GASTRIC SLEEVE BARIATRIC COOKBOOK FOR BEGINNERS

Nutrient-Dense Recipes For Post Surgery Recovery

Molly Maynard

Table of Contents

Introduction

Congratulations on taking the first step towards a healthier and happier life by undergoing gastric sleeve surgery. This cookbook is your essential companion as you embark on this transformative journey to better health and well-being.

We'll go over the basics of gastric sleeve surgery in this introduction, as well as how important nutrition is to your long-term success and post-surgical rehabilitation. In addition, we'll provide you insightful advice and pointers to assist you take advantage of the chances and overcome the difficulties presented by your new nutritional way of living.

A number of health issues, including comorbidities associated with obesity including diabetes, hypertension, and sleep apnea, can significantly improve after gastric sleeve surgery. It is an effective weight-loss technique. However, following surgery, success demands perseverance, commitment, and a readiness to adopt healthy dietary and lifestyle adjustments.

This cookbook offers delicious, nutritious, and simple-to-follow recipes that are customized to your specific dietary needs and constraints. It is specifically made for people who have had gastric sleeve surgery. These recipes will help you nourish your body, fuel your mind, and enjoy delectable meals that support your weight loss objectives. They range from protein-rich breakfasts to filling lunches and dinners, as well as decadent desserts and snacks.

Remind yourself that you are not alone as you start this new chapter in your life. This cookbook is meant to help and encourage you at every turn, to support you as you navigate the ups and downs, celebrate your victories, and get past any challenges that may come up—whether you're just starting out on your post-surgery journey or searching for new inspiration along the way.

Cheers to your well-being, joy, and fresh starts!

Chapter One

Understanding Gastric Sleeve Surgery

Sleeve gastrectomy, another name for gastric sleeve surgery, is a type of bariatric surgery. A large portion of your stomach is removed, leaving only a thin "sleeve." Your stomach becomes smaller, which aids in calorie restriction and suppresses hunger signals. For those who are clinically severe obese and want to lose weight effectively, this operation is offered.

What is gastric sleeve surgery?

The gastric sleeve, also referred to as a sleeve gastrectomy, is a bariatric surgery procedure intended to induce weight loss. It functions by making your stomach smaller. The removal of all or part of the stomach is known as a "gastrectomy". After a gastric sleeve procedure, around 80% of your stomach is removed, leaving behind a banana-sized, tubular "sleeve."

What does a gastric sleeve do?

Limiting your food intake in one sitting and experiencing satiety faster can be achieved by reducing your stomach.

But it also serves another purpose:

It minimizes the quantity of hunger hormones your stomach is capable of producing. This aids in reducing appetite and cravings and may help ward off the inclinations that lead people to regain weight they've lost.

Which medical issues can be treated with gastric sleeve surgery?

One surgical treatment for obesity and associated medical issues is gastric sleeve surgery. It is only available to qualified people who either already have significant obesity-related medical issues or are at high risk of developing them. Following gastric sleeve surgery, the following conditions may improve or perhaps go away:

- Insulin resistance and Type 2 diabetes.

- Hypertension and hypertensive heart disease.
- Hyperlipidemia (high cholesterol) and arterial disease.
- Nonalcoholic fatty liver disease and steatohepatitis.
- Obesity hypoventilation syndrome and obstructive sleep apnea.
- Joint pain and osteoarthritis.

Is the gastric sleeve safe?

Compared to the hazards of obesity and associated disorders, gastric sleeve surgery carries a significantly lower risk. Additionally, the complication rate is lower than that of other common operations, such as hip replacement and gallbladder surgery. The majority of gastric sleeve operations are carried out using minimally invasive surgical methods, which results in quicker recovery and reduced discomfort from incisions.

What qualifies you for gastric sleeve surgery?

To qualify, the general requirements are:

That you have severe obesity (class III). This is determined by your BMI (body mass index), which is calculated by your weight and height, and your related health conditions. A BMI of 40 or above, or a BMI of at least 35 along with at least one associated illness, is considered class III obesity.

That before the procedure, you attempted to lose weight but were unsuccessful. It can take up to six months to lose weight under a doctor's supervision before your insurance company will authorize and pay for the procedure.

That you are ready for the procedure and the recuperation period on a physical and mental level. You will have screening and counseling sessions with a group of dietitians, psychologists, and other medical professionals prior to being eligible for weight loss surgery.

What happens before gastric sleeve surgery?

Following your successful health exam and approval for bariatric sleeve surgery, you will embark on a two-week liquid diet. You will receive detailed instructions from your surgeon. To make the procedure safer, the goal is to reduce some of the fat in your liver and belly.

It is required of you to fast for 12 hours prior to your procedure. This is to guarantee that your stomach is empty throughout the process. Having food or liquid left in your stomach during the surgery could cause unpleasant or even dangerous side effects.

How is gastric sleeve surgery performed?

A sleeve gastrectomy is typically performed via robotic or laparoscopic surgery. That implies that your surgeon will execute the procedure through small incisions rather than making a major incision (or cut) to open your abdominal cavity and reach your organs. This facilitates a quicker recovery, however depending on their conditions, some patients can benefit more from open surgery.

What happens during gastric sleeve surgery?

You will be put to sleep during the procedure by your surgeon using general anesthetic.
Your surgeon will create a tiny, 1/2-inch-long cut in your belly and insert a port. To enlarge your abdomen, they will pump carbon dioxide gas via the port.
A tiny, illuminated video camera (laparoscope) will then be inserted into the port. Your interiors will be projected onto a screen by the camera.

Through one to three additional incisions, your surgeon will insert additional ports and complete the procedure using long, narrow tools.

Using a surgical stapler, they will divide and separate the remaining portion of your stomach after measuring out the gastric sleeve.

After removing the remaining stomach, your surgeon will seal your incisions.

How long does gastric sleeve surgery take?

A sleeve gastrectomy is a rather quick and straightforward process in comparison to other weight loss surgical methods.

It takes about 60 to 90 minutes. One to two days following the procedure, your surgeon might still want you to remain in the hospital. They can thus assist in treating your pain as well as any temporary surgical side effects, such nausea.

What happens after gastric sleeve surgery?

In the coming weeks and months, you will see your doctor frequently for check-ups. They'll keep an eye on your weight loss progress, any surgical side effects, and any related health issues. They'll also want to know if you're maintaining your weight loss and good health by taking good care of yourself and adhering to the required lifestyle guidelines.

After gastric sleeve surgery, will I have to follow a diet?

To ensure that your stomach heals properly, in the short term, you will need to adhere to stringent dietary restrictions. You may start eating a more normal diet after a few months, but you'll still need to make wise food choices. You will need to make sure that the food you do eat is nourishing enough to meet your energy demands because you won't be able to eat as much as before. Soon after surgery, you'll need to start taking vitamins, which you must do for the rest of your life.

What are the advantages of this procedure?

The gastric sleeve procedure is simpler, quicker, and safer than other bariatric surgery procedures. A sleeve gastrectomy is typically tolerable for patients with medical issues that may not be suitable for a longer procedure. Because the surgery doesn't rearrange your intestines, it's also much less likely to cause long-term complications related to nutrition.

Gastric sleeve gives good weight reduction and health benefits, however the typical weight loss is quite a bit lower than with more complex weight loss surgeries. Originally, this procedure was performed as the first of two steps of a bariatric procedure known as the duodenal switch. Surgeons started offering it as a standalone procedure after many people found that they didn't need to complete the second part.

What risks or complications could gastric sleeve surgery cause?

All surgeries have some risk of complications. With sleeve gastrectomy, they occur in less than 1% of operations. Surgical complications include:

- Bleeding.
- Infection.
- Reactions to anesthesia.
- Leaking from the staple line.

Some patients experience long-term surgical problems after they recuperate. When they do arise, they are typically simple to cure. They can include:

- **Scar tissue** after the operation can cause your stomach to be narrow, which can slow or block food from moving through your stomach causing nausea, vomiting, and difficulty eating.

- **Nutritional deficiencies**. Getting adequate nutrients is more difficult when you're eating a lot less. Following bariatric surgery, daily dietary supplements are typically prescribed for patients for the rest of their lives.

- **Gastroesophageal reflux**. Some people who did not have acid reflux prior to the procedure appear to develop it, and some who did believe that it worsens afterward. Medication is often an effective treatment for this.

- **Gallstones**. Gallstones may become more common if weight is lost quickly. It increases the amount of fat your liver processes, which can lead to cholesterol stones accumulating in your gallbladder and causing pain after meals. You may need another surgery to remove your gallbladder called a cholecystectomy.

How much time does recovery take following gastric sleeve surgery?

You should give yourself a good month before you expect to feel quite like yourself or return to work at full capacity. Many people experience fatigue or tiredness during this time while their bodies adjust to consuming less calories and heal. You will be able to handle only a liquid diet for the first few weeks. Over time, you'll gradually progress to a soft diet, and finally, solid foods.

With the gastric sleeve, how much weight will you lose?

The average weight loss is 25% to 30 % of your body weight in the first one to two years. In other words, you would drop 100 pounds if your starting weight was 300 pounds. Depending on your post-surgery habits, you may lose more or less. Some people also regain some weight, but the overall average weight loss of 25% to 30% of your body weight is consistent over five years.

What if it doesn't work?

While it isn't common, some people do regain the weight they lose. Over time, their stomach may expand again or they might go back to their old habits. You may want to think about having a gastric sleeve revision if this occurs to you. Your surgeon has two options: either fix the original gastric sleeve or switch it out for a more effective weight-loss procedure like a duodenal switch or gastric bypass.

Summary

A sleeve gastrectomy is an easy and safe surgery that can lead to significant weight loss. Furthermore, you will need to make lifelong adjustments because it will permanently alter your stomach. To protect your stomach and meet your nutritional needs, you will need to make extremely deliberate decisions about what and how you eat both after surgery and for the rest of your life.

But if you're committed to change and weight loss, surgery can help you be healthier. Not only does it limit your food intake, but it also lowers your blood sugar and decreases hunger, making eating fewer calories feel more natural. After having a gastric sleeve surgery, many obesity-related conditions can become better or perhaps go away.

Chapter Two

Importance Of Nutrition After Gastric Sleeve Surgery

Your eating habits will need to change following gastric sleeve surgery. Following surgery, the diet advances from a liquid to a pureed to a soft diet and finally to a modified diet. The goal of this process is to facilitate your body's healing. It's critical that you adhere to the eating plan in order to promote healing and reduce the likelihood of complications.

Pre-gastric sleeve diet

Reducing liver size is one of the primary dietary objectives prior to surgery. If you are obese, there is probably a buildup of fat cells in and around your liver. It is bigger than it ought to be because of this.

Your stomach and liver are situated next to each other. An enlarged liver makes gastric sleeve surgery more difficult for your doctor to perform and riskier for you to undergo.

You'll be given a specific diet to follow starting two weeks prior to the day of the surgery as preparation for the procedure.

It's a strict diet that cuts calories and carbs, which include pasta, potatoes, and sweets. Vegetables, low-or no-calorie beverages, and lean protein will be your main foods. It's possible that your doctor will give you a daily caloric goal to stick to.

You will go on a clear, liquid diet two days before surgery. This could involve drinking one low-sugar protein shake each day along with sugar-free popsicles, broth, water, and decaffeinated tea or coffee. Avoid carbonated and caffeine-infused drinks.

Why is weight loss required before surgery?

- To reduce body fat so that the surgeon can have better access, leading to safer surgery
- To make your liver smaller, which would otherwise be a hindrance

- Increased capacity to adjust to dietary requirements following surgery
- Shorter operating times and lower risks following surgery
- Enhanced mobility and physical function following surgery

Post-gastric sleeve diet

Week 1 diet

You will stick to the clear liquid diet you were on in the days before surgery for the first week following the surgery.

This will lessen the chance of postoperative complications including dehydration, diarrhea, constipation, gastric leakage, and bowel blockage. This regimen will assist your body in healing over the course of time that it needs. Certain things to bear in mind are:

- Drink lots of clear drinks. See your doctor about electrolyte beverages to try, such as calorie-free Gatorade, if you struggle to stay hydrated.

- Stay away from sugar-filled beverages. Dumping syndrome is a medical condition that arises when the small intestine is rapidly overflowed with sugar. As a result, there is extreme fatigue, nausea, diarrhea, and possibly vomiting. Sugar also has a lot of empty calories. it should be avoided for now and minimized over time.

- Caffeine should be avoided since it may aggravate acid reflux and dehydration.

- Gas and bloating can be caused by carbonated drinks, such as sugar-filled ones, calorie-free choices, and seltzer. After surgery, and maybe even in the long run, all of these should be avoided.

Week 2 diet

You'll transition to a full-liquid diet during the second week following the procedure. Options consist of:

- No-sugar nutrition shakes, such as Ensure Light
- Instant breakfast drinks
- Shakes made with protein powder

- thin broth and cream-based soups with no chunks — soft soup noodles are ok in very small amounts
- Unsweetened milk
- Sugar-free, nonfat pudding
- Ice cream, sorbet, and sugar-free, nonfat frozen yogurt
- Nonfat plain Greek yogurt
- Fruit juices diluted with water, with no pulp
- Oatmeal or hot cereal that has been thinned out, like Cream of Wheat

Your appetite could seem to be increasing during this time. While it's entirely normal, that doesn't mean you should eat solid food. You still can't manage solids in your system. Vomiting and other complications can result.

Drinking lots of liquids and staying away from sugar and fat will help you get ready for the next phase of your diet. Carbonated beverages and caffeine should still be avoided.

Week 3 diet

You can start including soft, pureed foods in your diet during the third week. Eat mindfully and properly chew your food—at least 25 times, if you can. Anything you can purée that is low in fat and sugar is OK, such as nonfibrous veggies and lean protein sources.

It's critical to begin consuming more protein. If you find pureed lean protein sources too bland, stick to eating eggs every day or drinking protein shakes without added sugar.
Foods to eat include:
- Jarred baby food
- Silken tofu
- Cooked, pureed white fish
- Soft-scrambled or soft-boiled eggs
- Soup
- Cottage cheese
- Canned fruit in juice
- Mashed bananas or very ripe mango
- Hummus
- Pureed or mashed avocado
- Plain Greek yogurt

During this period, avoid solid, chunky foods as well as caffeine. Additionally, you should stick to plain foods with minimal or no seasoning. Spices may contribute to heartburn.

Week 4 diet

You can start incorporating solid foods into your diet now that you've had surgery for one month.

Now is the perfect moment to fully implement your newly acquired knowledge about healthy eating. Hard-to-digest meals like steak, fibrous vegetables, and nuts should still be avoided, as should sugar, oil, and high-fat dairy products.

Other items to stay away from are white potatoes, pasta, and other high-carb foods. During this period, caffeine-containing beverages can typically be reintroduced in moderation. Below are foods you can add to your list:

- Well-cooked chicken and fish
- Well-cooked vegetables
- Sweet potatoes
- Low-fat cheese
- Fruit
- Low-sugar cereal

Week 5 Diet and beyond

Now that you may safely eat solid food, it's time to implement your new, normal eating plan for the long term. Lean protein and veggies should be the main focus. Introduce foods one at a time so you can keep an eye on how your body reacts.

Foods like soda and sugary sweets are something you should either completely avoid or limit your intake of going forward. You can resume eating any other foods as long as they don't cause any problems.

Make sensible dietary choices by avoiding empty calories and selecting nutrient-dense foods. Maintaining your diet may be made easier if you eat three small meals and few snacks each day. Additionally, remember to stay hydrated at all times.

Guidelines and tips

Here are some post-surgery healing pointers to help you stay on course:

- Use a blender or food processor to purée food.
- Understand the difference between appetite (mental/emotional) and hunger (physical).
- Don't overeat — over time, the size of your stomach will expand and stabilize.
- Chew slowly, and eat slowly.
- Avoid non-nutrient calories.
- Avoid concentrated sugars.
- Avoid trans fats and fried, processed, and fast foods.
- Drink water or low-calorie Gatorade to prevent dehydration.

- Avoid consuming food and liquids simultaneously.
-
- To determine what you should take and when, discuss bariatric vitamins and supplements with your doctor.
- Build movement into your life. Start with walking, and explore other exercises that you enjoy, such as swimming, dancing, and yoga.
- Avoid alcohol. Other bariatric procedures, including gastric sleeve surgery, may intensify and accelerate the effects of alcohol.
- Avoid nonsteroidal anti-inflammatory drugs (NSAIDs), such as Ibuprofen, aspirin, and naproxen. These kinds of over-the-counter painkillers might decrease the natural coating that protects your stomach.

It's crucial that you adhere to the eating plan your doctor prescribes for you prior to and following gastric sleeve surgery. The foods that you are permitted to eat are intended to support both your body's healing process and the development of a lifelong healthy eating habit. Exercise is also a vitally important element.

Chapter Three

Preparing for Your Gastric Sleeve journey

A weight loss surgery is a big life decision that needs to be planned and thought through. An option that is becoming more and more popular for people seeking bariatric surgery to reduce a significant amount of weight is gastric sleeve surgery. There are alternatives for a surgical revision if you gain weight after a gastric sleeve.

It is imperative that you begin your preparations for gastric sleeve surgery as soon as possible if you are considering the procedure. As this kind of surgery is a major life change, there are steps you may take to get ready, both mentally and physically.

Mental Preparation for Gastric Sleeve Surgery

Being mentally and emotionally ready is essential before having a sleeve gastrectomy or any other bariatric treatment. The physical implications of the operation coupled with the major lifestyle changes might be overwhelming. Here's how to get ready emotionally and mentally for this life-changing event:

Comprehensive Conversations with Your Operating Doctor

- **Understanding Risks:** Talk in-depth about the specific risks connected to sleeve gastrectomy, including any personal health issues that may affect these risks.

- **Procedure Selection:** Find out which bariatric operation best fits your lifestyle, health, and weight loss objectives.

- **Safety Measures:** To guarantee your safety, find out what precautions are taken before, during, and after the procedure.

- **Preparation and Recovery:** Learn everything there is to know about the recovery process and how to get ready for the procedure.

Engaging with Patient Stories and Community Resources

- **Research:** Take in patient stories, watch documentaries, and read articles to gain a comprehensive understanding of the adventure you are about to embark on.

- **Communities and Forums:** Participate in social media groups or forums devoted to bariatric surgery to hear from others who have been through the procedure and exchange experiences.

- **Direct Conversations:** Try to get in touch with people who have had the surgery directly to learn about their successes, difficulties, and experiences.

- **Notify Important Parties:** Tell your loved ones, friends, and coworkers about your plans and how they may help you during this time.

- **Professional Support:** Speak with a therapist or counselor who specializes in guiding people through bariatric surgery and the corresponding lifestyle modifications. Any underlying problems with eating, stress, and body image may be helped by this.

Understanding Complications and Recovery

- **Recognizing Symptoms:** Learn the differences between common as well as rare complications, how to identify them, and when to consult a doctor.

- **Managing Expectations:** Recognize the typical indicators of recovery so you can distinguish between typical post-operative discomfort and indications of complications.

Psychological Readiness

- **Mental Health Assessment:** Talking with a mental health professional can help you develop coping mechanisms for the psychological and emotional difficulties that come with this transformative experience.

- **Stress Management:** Realize that stress can affect the results of weight loss and healing, so learn stress-reduction strategies that work for you.

- **Emotional resilience:** To successfully navigate the highs and lows of the post-surgery journey, including probable setbacks in weight loss or health improvements, it is imperative to develop emotional resilience.

Preparing for Long-term Weight Loss Success

There are crucial steps you must not miss if you want to ensure that your weight loss will continue for up to ten years following your gastric sleeve surgery.

- **Lifestyle Modifications:** Accept that surgery is a tool that necessitates substantial and long-term lifestyle modifications rather than a quick fix.

- **Commitment to Follow-Up:** To guarantee the greatest results, make a commitment to the required follow-up consultations, dietary recommendations, and exercise regimens.

In addition to giving you a clearer mental state throughout the procedure, this all-encompassing approach to mental and emotional preparation can greatly improve your chances of long-term success and lifestyle adjustment.

Physical activity

It is advised to begin or maintain an exercise regimen prior to surgery. By increasing your level of fitness, you can make the procedure safer and your recuperation go more smoothly. Make sure your physical activity is appropriate for your current level of fitness, and before beginning any new fitness regimen, always get advice from your healthcare professional.

Understanding Nutritional Needs Post-Surgery

It is imperative that you familiarize yourself with the post-operative nutritional phases. You will go from a liquid diet to pureed foods and finally to solid foods following surgery. It is crucial for your long-term health and recuperation to understand your future nutritional regimen, including the significance of vitamin and mineral supplements and maintaining hydration.

Lifestyle Adjustments and Support Systems

Long-term lifestyle adjustments are required to sustain weight loss and enhance health. This entails maintaining a healthy diet and engaging in frequent exercise. Strong support networks, whether made up of friends, family, support groups, or counseling, can offer the accountability and encouragement required to stick to these adjustments.

Pre-Surgical Logistics

Making transportation arrangements, packing for the hospital, and being aware of the kind of care you'll require at home while recovering are all important practical preparations for the day of surgery. It's crucial to schedule time off work and help with domestic chores while you recover.

Final Consultation with the Surgical Team

You get the chance to verify that you understand the operation, risks, advantages, and post-operative care plan during your final pre-operative appointment. This is the ideal opportunity to address any last-minute queries or worries.

It is essential to prepare for your sleeve gastrectomy in order to have a successful procedure and long-term health benefits. A healthier future is put in motion when pre-operative preparation is actively participated in.

Chapter Four

Stocking Your Kitchen with Essentials

Many bariatric patients clear out harmful items from their cupboards in order to resist temptations. But while junk food is simple to spot, bariatric patients might not know how to stock their cabinets with healthier alternatives. After weight loss surgery, pantry essentials have a new significance to suit your new dietary requirements.

To make sure you're adhering to your pre- or post-operative diet and avoiding temptation, it's crucial to keep your pantry and refrigerator well-stocked with nutritious foods.

You can find nutritious snacks easily, make bariatric-friendly meals with ease, and enhance your protein consumption by keeping the following supplies on hand:

Here are a few staples to stock up on:

- **Canned Tuna/Salmon/Chicken** - These are high in protein and very convenient. Toss them over a green salad or pair them with sliced vegetables.

- **Snacks** - Look for snacks that are high in fiber and protein, low in calories, and low in added sugar. Nuts such as almonds are an excellent option.

- **Protein Bars** - Protein bars are a convenient option for a fast meal on the go. Just be cautious—certain components have a tendency to be heavy in sugar.

- **Unflavored whey protein** - You'll likely drink a lot of protein shakes during the liquid-diet phase of your surgery recovery, but protein powder goes well in many other foods and beverages. However, protein powders come in a variety of flavors, and you may not always want to add a vanilla or chocolate punch to your food. Unflavored whey protein is a great way to increase your protein without affecting the flavor of what you're eating. For instance, you can add unflavored whey protein powder to soup or Greek yogurt.

- **Poultry, Beef and Plant-Based Protein Sources** - Store your preferred lean meat cuts in the freezer and defrost them when you're ready to prepare a high-protein meal.

  Some favorites include chicken breast, ground turkey and lean ground beef. Check the components when selecting plant-based protein sources, such as veggie burgers. Two excellent plant-based protein sources are tofu and beans.

- **Low-Carb Wraps** - These are a nutritious option for tacos or sandwiches.

- **Salmon** - As a great source of omega-3s and protein, salmon is a healthy food staple. When buying frozen salmon, most of it come in individually wrapped filets, which makes it easy to defrost the portions you need.

- **Frozen Vegetables** - Stock up on your favorite frozen veggies, such as broccoli, asparagus, peppers, cauliflower, and more, to go with your preferred protein for a nutritious and bariatric-friendly meal.

- **Frozen Fruit** - Combine with protein powder, skim milk, or unsweetened almond milk in smoothies. When choosing fruit, stick to berries (strawberries, blueberries, blackberries, and raspberries) as they contain less sugar than other types of fruit.

- **Greek yogurt** - A high-protein, healthful breakfast choice. Check the ingredients and select the variety with higher protein and less sugar.

- **Eggs** - Eggs make a tasty breakfast option. You can meal prep as egg muffins, quiche or even hard boil them

- **Milk** - If you're choosing a non-dairy milk, go for the unsweetened version.

- **Cheese** - Low fat cheese sticks or reduced fat cheeses make great snacks to take on the go

- **Salads** - Choose spring mix for salads and include raw veggies like tomatoes, peppers, and cucumbers.

- **Powdered peanut butter** - Compared to standard peanut butter, powdered peanut butter has less fat and calories and offers about the same amount of protein. For instance, two tablespoons of PB2 have 60 calories, 1.5 g of fat, 2 g of sugar, and 6 g of protein. Another excellent choice is PBfit, which has 70 calories, 2g fat, 2g sugar, and 8g protein in every two tablespoons. Standard peanut butter, on the other hand, contains 190 calories, 16g fat, 3g sugar, and 7g protein. Using a peanut butter powder instead of a traditional spread is around one-third of the calories and cuts your fat intake by up to 90%.

- **Sugar substitute** - After bariatric surgery, you don't have to give up on baked goods. There are a ton of protein-rich muffins, cupcakes, and other recipe options available online. To cut calories and sugar intake, is a must to use a sugar substitute; a little goes a long way. For instance, the sweetness of half a teaspoon of stevia sugar substitute is equal to that of one cup of sugar. However, stevia has zero calories and carbohydrates compared to sugar's 773 calories and 200g of carbohydrates.

Keeping basic, healthful food alternatives stocked in your pantry makes sticking to your bariatric diet much easier. Another important strategy for avoiding boredom and diet dissatisfaction is variety.

Post Bariatric Surgery Meal Plan Guidelines

It is important to follow certain meal planning guidelines after bariatric surgery to promote weight loss:

- Stick to 3 small meals and 2 bariatric friendly snacks per day. For patients to maintain optimal blood sugar levels, they should eat roughly every three hours. Small, frequent meals also prevent overeating.

- Focus on protein at each meal. A daily intake of 70–90g of protein aids in maintaining muscle mass during periods of rapid weight loss. Lean meats, salmon, tuna, eggs, Greek yogurt, cottage cheese, and chicken breast are all excellent sources of protein. High-protein meal substitutes, such as the finest bariatric protein shakes and snacks, can also be included.

- Keep carbohydrates to 1/4 of the plate and prioritize non-starchy veggies. Starchy foods like grains, breads, pasta, and rice can hinder weight loss. To add volume and nutrients, fill half of the plate with low-carb vegetables. Broccoli, cauliflower, carrots, peppers, green beans, and leafy greens are all excellent options.

- Drink 64 ounces or more of fluids a day to stay hydrated. Dehydration can be avoided with a diet rich in low-calorie drinks like broth, unsweetened tea, and enough water. Additionally, fluids facilitate digestion and ward off constipation.

- Avoid high fat, high sugar foods. These calorie-dense foods can slow weight loss. Opt for bariatric foods such as low-fat dairy, lean proteins, whole grains, and produce. Limit added sugars, fried items, heavy sauces, and sweet treats.

- Take vitamins and supplements as recommended. Certain nutrients may be more difficult to absorb after bariatric surgery. Daily vitamin and mineral recommendations from doctors help to prevent dietary deficits. Bariatric multivitamins, calcium, iron, vitamin B12, and vitamin D are examples of common supplements.

Chapter Five

Clear liquid recipes

Here are clear liquid recipes suitable for the initial stage after gastric sleeve surgery:

Chicken Broth

Ingredients:

- 2 cups water
- 1 chicken bouillon cube or 1 teaspoon chicken bouillon powder

Preparation:

- Boil water in a saucepan.

- Add the chicken bouillon cube or powder and stir until dissolved.

- Simmer for a few minutes.

- Take out from the heat and let it cool slightly before serving.

Cooking Time: 5 minutes

Number of Servings: 2

Nutritional Information (per serving):

- Calories: 5
- Protein: 1g
- Carbohydrates: 0g
- Fat: 0g

Sugar-Free Gelatin

Ingredients:

- 1 package sugar-free gelatin mix
- 2 cups boiling water

Preparation:

- In a heatproof bowl, dissolve the sugar-free gelatin mix in boiling water.

- Stir until completely dissolved.

- Pour the mixture into individual serving cups.

- Refrigerate until set, usually about 2 hours.

Cooking Time: 2 hours (setting time)

Number of Servings: 4

Nutritional Information (per serving):

- Calories: 5
- Protein: 1g
- Carbohydrates: 0g
- Fat: 0g

Clear Vegetable Broth

Ingredients:

- 2 cups water
- 1 vegetable bouillon cube or 1 teaspoon vegetable bouillon powder
- 1/2 carrot, peeled and chopped
- 1 celery stalk, chopped
- 1/2 onion, peeled and chopped
- Salt and pepper to taste

Preparation:

- Boil water in a saucepan.

- Add the vegetable bouillon cube or powder and stir until dissolved.

- Add chopped carrot, celery, and onion to the boiling water.

- For 10-15 minutes, simmer the vegetables until they are soft.

- Strain the broth to remove the vegetables.

- For taste, season with salt and pepper before serving.

Cooking Time: 15 minutes

Number of Servings: 2

Nutritional Information (per serving):

- Calories: 10
- Protein: 1g
- Carbohydrates: 2g
- Fat: 0g

Herbal Tea

Ingredients:

- 1 herbal tea bag (like chamomile, peppermint, or ginger)
- 1 cup boiling water

Preparation:

- Place the herbal tea bag in a mug.

- Pour boiling water over the tea bag.

- Let it steep for 5-7 minutes.

- Remove the tea bag and discard.

- Before drinking, allow the tea to cool slightly.

Preparation Time: 5-7 minutes

Number of Servings: 1

Nutritional Information (per serving):

- Calories: 0
- Protein: 0g

- Carbohydrates: 0g
- Fat: 0g

Beef Broth

Ingredients:

- 2 cups water
- 1 beef bouillon cube or 1 teaspoon beef bouillon powder

Preparation:

- Boil water in a saucepan.

- Add the beef bouillon cube or powder and stir until dissolved.

- Simmer for a few minutes.

- Take out from the heat and let it cool slightly before serving.

Preparation Time: 5 minutes

Number of Servings: 2

Nutritional Information (per serving):

- Calories: 5
- Protein: 1g
- Carbohydrates: 0g
- Fat: 0g

Apple Juice Gelatin

Ingredients:

- 1 package sugar-free apple-flavored gelatin mix
- 1 1/2 cups boiling water
- 1/2 cup unsweetened apple juice

Preparation:

- In a heatproof bowl, dissolve the sugar-free apple-flavored gelatin mix in boiling water.

- Stir until completely dissolved.

- Add unsweetened apple juice to the mixture and stir until combined.

- Pour the mixture into individual serving cups.

- Refrigerate until set, usually about 2 hours.

Preparation Time: 2 hours (setting time)

Number of Servings: 4

Nutritional Information (per serving):

- Calories: 5
- Protein: 1g
- Carbohydrates: 0g
- Fat: 0g

Lemonade Ice Pops

Ingredients:

- 1 cup water
- 2 tablespoons lemon juice
- 1 tablespoon sugar or sugar substitute

Preparation:

- In a bowl, mix together water, lemon juice, and sugar until sugar is dissolved.

- Turn the mixture into ice pop molds.

- Insert ice pop sticks and freeze until solid, usually about 4-6 hours.

Preparation Time: 5 minutes (plus freezing time)

Number of Servings: 4 ice pops

Nutritional Information (per serving):

- Calories: 5
- Protein: 0g
- Carbohydrates: 1g
- Fat: 0g

Clear Chicken Consommé

Ingredients:

- 4 cups chicken broth (low-sodium)
- 2 egg whites
- 1/4 cup cold water
- Salt and pepper to taste

Preparation:

- In a saucepan, heat the chicken broth until hot but not boiling.

- In a bowl, whisk together egg whites and cold water until frothy.

- Slowly pour the egg white mixture into the hot chicken broth while stirring gently.

- Continue to cook over low heat, stirring occasionally, until the egg whites form a raft on top.

- Carefully ladle the clear consommé through a fine mesh sieve to remove the egg whites.

- For taste, season with salt and pepper before serving.

Preparation Time: 15 minutes

Number of Servings: 4

Nutritional Information (per serving):

- Calories: 10
- Protein: 2g
- Carbohydrates: 0g
- Fat: 0g

During the early phases following gastric sleeve surgery, these clear liquid recipes are easy on the stomach and offer hydration and some essential nutrients. Based on your nutritional requirements and tastes, modify the portion sizes and ingredients.

For personalized guidance, speak with a dietician or your healthcare professional.

Chapter Six

Full liquid recipes

Here are full liquid recipes suitable for the next stage after clear liquids, typically during the recovery period after gastric sleeve surgery:

Protein Shake

Ingredients:

- 1 scoop protein powder (whey or plant-based)
- 1 cup of milk (skim milk or unsweetened almond milk)
- 1/2 banana or other fruit (optional)
- Ice cubes

Preparation:

- In a blender, combine protein powder, almond milk, fruit (if using), and ice cubes.

- Blend until smooth and creamy.

- Pour into a glass and serve immediately.

Number of Servings: 1

Nutritional Information (per serving):

- Calories: 200-250 (depending on protein powder and additions)
- Protein: 20-25g
- Carbohydrates: 15-20g
- Fat: 5-10g

Creamy Tomato Soup

Ingredients:

- 1 cup tomato soup (low-sodium)
- 1/2 cup of milk (skim milk or unsweetened almond milk)
- Salt and pepper to taste
- Fresh basil leaves for garnish (optional)

Preparation:

- In a saucepan, heat tomato soup over medium heat.

- Stir in almond milk or skim milk until well combined.

- Season with salt and pepper to taste.

- If desired, before serving, garnish with fresh basil leaves.

Number of Servings: 1

Nutritional Information (per serving):

- Calories: 100-150 (depending on type of soup and milk used)
- Protein: 3-5g
- Carbohydrates: 15-20g
- Fat: 3-5g

Vanilla Yogurt Smoothie

Ingredients:

- 1/2 cup plain Greek yogurt
- 1/2 cup of milk (skim milk or unsweetened almond milk)
- 1/2 teaspoon vanilla extract
- 1/2 tablespoon honey or maple syrup (optional)
- Ice cubes

Preparation:

- In a blender, combine Greek yogurt, almond milk, vanilla extract, honey or maple syrup (if using), and ice cubes.

- Blend until smooth and creamy.

- Pour into a glass and serve immediately.

Number of Servings: 1

Nutritional Information (per serving):

- Calories: 150-200 (depending on type of yogurt and additions)
- Protein: 10-15g
- Carbohydrates: 15-20g
- Fat: 5-7g

Chocolate Avocado Pudding

Ingredients:

- 1 ripe avocado
- 2 tablespoons unsweetened cocoa powder
- 2 tablespoons honey or maple syrup
- 1/4 cup of milk (skim milk or unsweetened almond milk)

- Dash of vanilla extract

Preparation:

- In a blender or food processor, combine avocado, cocoa powder, honey or maple syrup, almond milk, and vanilla extract.

- Blend until smooth and creamy.

- Transfer it to a bowl or individual serving cups.

- Before serving, chill in the refrigerator for at least 30 minutes.

Number of Servings: 2

Nutritional Information (per serving):

- Calories: 150-200 (depending on sweetener used)
- Protein: 2-3g
- Carbohydrates: 15-20g
- Fat: 10-15g

Banana Coconut Smoothie

Ingredients:

- 1 ripe banana
- 1/2 cup coconut milk
- 1/2 cup of milk (skim milk or unsweetened almond milk)
- 1 tablespoon shredded coconut (unsweetened)
- Ice cubes

Preparation:

- In a blender, combine banana, coconut milk, almond milk, shredded coconut, and ice cubes.

- Blend until smooth and creamy.

- Pour into a glass and serve immediately.

Number of Servings: 1

Nutritional Information (per serving):

- Calories: 200-250
- Protein: 2-3g
- Carbohydrates: 25-30g

- Fat: 10-15g

Strawberry Banana Protein Smoothie

Ingredients:

- 1/2 cup frozen strawberries
- 1/2 banana
- 1 scoop vanilla protein powder
- 1/2 cup of milk (skim milk or unsweetened almond milk)
- Ice cubes

Preparation:

- In a blender, combine frozen strawberries, banana, vanilla protein powder, almond milk, and ice cubes.

- Blend until smooth and creamy.

- Pour into a glass and serve immediately.

Number of Servings: 1

Nutritional Information (per serving):

- Calories: 200-250
- Protein: 20-25g

- Carbohydrates: 25-30g
- Fat: 5-7g

Creamy Peanut Butter Shake

Ingredients:

- 1 tablespoon natural peanut butter
- 1 scoop chocolate protein powder
- 1/2 cup of milk (skim milk or unsweetened almond milk)
- Ice cubes

Preparation:

- In a blender, combine peanut butter, chocolate protein powder, almond milk, and ice cubes.

- Blend until smooth and creamy.

- Pour into a glass and serve immediately.

Number of Servings: 1

Nutritional Information (per serving):

- Calories: 250-300
- Protein: 25-30g

- Carbohydrates: 10-15g
- Fat: 10-15g

Creamy Carrot Soup

Ingredients:

- 1 cup cooked carrots
- 1 cup vegetable or chicken broth
- 1/4 cup of milk (skim milk or unsweetened almond milk)
- Salt and pepper to taste

Preparation:

- In a blender, combine cooked carrots, broth, almond milk, salt, and pepper.

- Blend until smooth.

- Transfer the mixture to a saucepan.

- Heat the mixture over medium heat until thoroughly warmed.

- Serve hot.

Number of Servings: 1

Nutritional Information (per serving):

- Calories: 100-150
- Protein: 2-3g
- Carbohydrates: 15-20g
- Fat: 3-5g

Vanilla Coconut Milkshake

Ingredients:

- 1 cup coconut milk
- 1 scoop vanilla protein powder
- 1/2 teaspoon vanilla extract
- Ice cubes

Preparation:

- In a blender, combine coconut milk, vanilla protein powder, vanilla extract, and ice cubes.

- Blend until smooth and creamy.

- Pour into a glass and serve immediately.

Number of Servings: 1

Nutritional Information (per serving):

- Calories: 200-250
- Protein: 20-25g
- Carbohydrates: 5-10g
- Fat: 10-15g

Avocado Green Smoothie

Ingredients:

- 1/2 ripe avocado
- 1 cup spinach leaves
- 1/2 cup of milk (skim milk or unsweetened almond milk)
- 1 tablespoon honey or maple syrup (optional)
- Ice cubes

Preparation:

- In a blender, combine avocado, spinach leaves, almond milk, honey or maple syrup (if using), and ice cubes.

- Blend until smooth and creamy.

- Pour into a glass and serve immediately.

Number of Servings: 1

Nutritional Information (per serving):

- Calories: 200-250
- Protein: 5-10g
- Carbohydrates: 15-20g
- Fat: 15-20g

Following gastric sleeve surgery, these comprehensive liquid recipes offer nutrients and variety during the healing phase. To suit your nutritional requirements and preferences, modify the ingredients and portion sizes. For personalized guidance, speak with a dietician or your healthcare professional.

Chapter Seven

Pureed recipes

Here are pureed recipes suitable for the stage after full liquids, typically during the recovery period after gastric sleeve surgery:

Butternut Squash Soup

Ingredients:

- 2 cups cooked butternut squash
- 1 cup vegetable or chicken broth
- 1/2 cup of milk (skim milk or unsweetened almond milk)
- 1/4 teaspoon ground nutmeg
- Salt and pepper to taste

Preparation:

- In a blender, combine cooked butternut squash, broth, almond milk, nutmeg, salt, and pepper.

- Blend until smooth.

- The mixture should be transferred to a saucepan and heat over medium heat until warmed through.

- Serve hot.

Number of Servings: 2

Nutritional Information (per serving):

- Calories: 100-150
- Protein: 2-3g
- Carbohydrates: 20-25g
- Fat: 2-3g

Creamy Spinach and Ricotta Pasta

Ingredients:

- 1 cup cooked pasta (penne or rotini)
- 1 cup cooked spinach
- 1/2 cup ricotta cheese
- 1/4 cup of milk (skim milk or unsweetened almond milk)
- Garlic powder, salt, and pepper to taste

Preparation:

- In a blender, combine cooked pasta, cooked spinach, ricotta cheese, almond milk, garlic powder, salt, and pepper.

- Blend until smooth.

- The mixture should be transferred to a saucepan and heat over medium heat until warmed through.

- Serve warm.

Number of Servings: 2

Nutritional Information (per serving):

- Calories: 200-250
- Protein: 10-15g
- Carbohydrates: 20-25g
- Fat: 8-10g

Turkey and Vegetable Puree

Ingredients:

- 1/2 cup cooked turkey breast

- 1/2 cup cooked vegetables (carrots, peas, and green beans)
- 1/4 cup low-sodium chicken broth
- 1/4 cup of milk (skim milk or unsweetened almond milk)
- Salt and pepper to taste

Preparation:

- In a blender, combine cooked turkey breast, cooked vegetables, chicken broth, almond milk, salt, and pepper.

- Blend until smooth.

- The mixture should be transferred to a saucepan and heat over medium heat until warmed through.

- Serve warm.

Number of Servings: 1

Nutritional Information (per serving):

- Calories: 150-200
- Protein: 20-25g
- Carbohydrates: 10-15g
- Fat: 5-8g

Creamy Cauliflower Mash

Ingredients:

- 2 cups cooked cauliflower florets
- 1/4 cup low-fat cream cheese
- 1/4 cup of milk (skim milk or unsweetened almond milk)
- 1 tablespoon butter or olive oil
- Salt and pepper to taste

Preparation:

- In a blender, combine cooked cauliflower florets, cream cheese, almond milk, butter or olive oil, salt, and pepper.

- Blend until smooth.

- The mixture should be transferred to a saucepan and heat over medium heat until warmed through.

- Serve warm.

Number of Servings: 2

Nutritional Information (per serving):

- Calories: 100-150
- Protein: 5-7g
- Carbohydrates: 10-15g
- Fat: 5-8g

Creamy Chicken and Potato Puree

Ingredients:

- 1/2 cup cooked chicken breast
- 1/2 cup cooked potato
- 1/4 cup low-sodium chicken broth
- 1/4 cup of milk (skim milk or unsweetened almond milk)
- Salt and pepper to taste

Preparation:

- In a blender, combine cooked chicken breast, cooked potato, chicken broth, almond milk, salt, and pepper.

- Blend until smooth.

- The mixture should be transferred to a saucepan and heat over medium heat until warmed through.

- Serve warm.

Number of Servings: 1

Nutritional Information (per serving):

- Calories: 150-200
- Protein: 20-25g
- Carbohydrates: 10-15g
- Fat: 5-8g

Creamy Broccoli Soup

Ingredients:

- 1 cup cooked broccoli florets
- 1 cup vegetable or chicken broth
- 1/4 cup of milk (skim milk or unsweetened almond milk)
- 1 tablespoon low-fat cream cheese
- Salt and pepper to taste

Preparation:

- In a blender, combine cooked broccoli florets, broth, almond milk, cream cheese, salt, and pepper.

- Blend until smooth.

- The mixture should be transferred to a saucepan and heat over medium heat until warmed through.

- Serve hot.

Number of Servings: 2

Nutritional Information (per serving):

- Calories: 100-150
- Protein: 5-7g
- Carbohydrates: 10-15g
- Fat: 4-6g

Creamy Lentil Soup

Ingredients:

- 1/2 cup cooked lentils
- 1 cup vegetable or chicken broth
- 1/4 cup of milk (skim milk or unsweetened almond milk)
- 1/4 teaspoon ground cumin
- Salt and pepper to taste

Preparation:

- In a blender, combine cooked lentils, broth, almond milk, ground cumin, salt, and pepper.

- Blend until smooth.

- The mixture should be transferred to a saucepan and heat over medium heat until warmed through.

- Serve hot.

Number of Servings: 1

Nutritional Information (per serving):

- Calories: 150-200
- Protein: 10-15g
- Carbohydrates: 20-25g
- Fat: 3-5g

Creamy Mushroom Puree

Ingredients:

- 1 cup cooked mushrooms
- 1/2 cup vegetable or chicken broth

- 1/4 cup of milk (skim milk or unsweetened almond milk)
- 1 tablespoon low-fat cream cheese
- Salt and pepper to taste

Preparation:

- In a blender, combine cooked mushrooms, broth, almond milk, cream cheese, salt, and pepper.

- Blend until smooth.

- The mixture should be transferred to a saucepan and heat over medium heat until warmed through.

- Serve warm.

Number of Servings: 2

Nutritional Information (per serving):

- Calories: 100-150
- Protein: 5-7g
- Carbohydrates: 10-15g
- Fat: 4-6g

Creamy Pumpkin Soup

Ingredients:

- 1 cup canned pumpkin puree
- 1 cup vegetable or chicken broth
- 1/4 cup of milk (skim milk or unsweetened almond milk)
- 1/2 teaspoon ground cinnamon
- Salt and pepper to taste

Preparation:

- In a blender, combine canned pumpkin puree, broth, almond milk, ground cinnamon, salt, and pepper.

- Blend until smooth.

- The mixture should be transferred to a saucepan and heat over medium heat until warmed through.

- Serve hot.

Number of Servings: 2

Nutritional Information (per serving):

- Calories: 100-150
- Protein: 2-3g
- Carbohydrates: 20-25g
- Fat: 2-3g

Creamy Cauliflower and Leek Soup

Ingredients:

- 1 cup cooked cauliflower florets
- 1/2 cup cooked leeks
- 1 cup vegetable or chicken broth
- 1/4 cup of milk (skim milk or unsweetened almond milk)
- Salt and pepper to taste

Preparation:

- In a blender, combine cooked cauliflower florets, cooked leeks, broth, almond milk, salt, and pepper.

- Blend until smooth.

- The mixture should be transferred to a saucepan and heat over medium heat until warmed through.

- Serve hot.

Number of Servings: 2

Nutritional Information (per serving):

- Calories: 100-150
- Protein: 3-5g
- Carbohydrates: 15-20g
- Fat: 3-5g

Following gastric sleeve surgery, these pureed recipes provide a range of flavors and nutrients to aid with your recovery. For personalized nutritional guidance, speak with your healthcare professional or dietician and make any necessary adjustments to the ingredients and portion sizes.

Chapter Eight

Gastric Sleeve-Friendly Breakfast Recipes

Protein-Packed Greek Yogurt Parfait

Ingredients:

- 1 cup non-fat or low-fat plain Greek yogurt
- 1/4 cup fresh berries (strawberries, blueberries, or raspberries)
- 1 tablespoon chia seeds
- 1 tablespoon sliced almonds
- 1 teaspoon honey (optional)

Preparation:

- Spoon the Greek yogurt into a bowl or parfait glass.

- Layer with fresh berries on top of the yogurt.

- Sprinkle chia seeds and sliced almonds over the berries.

- Drizzle with honey if desired for extra sweetness.

Cooking Time: 5 minutes

Number of Servings: 1

Nutritional Information:

- Calories: 200
- Protein: 20g
- Carbohydrates: 18g
- Fiber: 5g
- Fat: 7g

Veggie and Egg White Omelette

Ingredients:

- 4 egg whites
- 1/4 cup chopped spinach
- 1/4 cup diced bell pepper
- 1/4 cup diced tomatoes
- 1 tablespoon low-fat feta cheese (optional)
- Salt and pepper to taste
- Cooking spray or 1 teaspoon olive oil

Preparation:

- Spray a non-stick skillet with cooking spray or add olive oil and heat over medium heat.

- Add the diced bell pepper and tomatoes, and sauté for 2-3 minutes until softened.

- Add the chopped spinach and cook for another 1-2 minutes until wilted.

- Pour in the egg whites and cook, stirring occasionally, until the eggs are fully cooked.

- Season with salt and pepper to taste.

- Optional: sprinkle with low-fat feta cheese before serving.

Cooking Time: 10 minutes

Number of Servings: 1

Nutritional Information:

- Calories: 120
- Protein: 20g
- Carbohydrates: 5g

- Fiber: 2g
- Fat: 2g

Cottage Cheese and Berry Bowl

Ingredients:

- 1 cup low-fat cottage cheese
- 1/2 cup mixed berries (blueberries, strawberries, raspberries)
- 1 tablespoon ground flaxseed
- 1 teaspoon honey (optional)

Preparation:

- Place the cottage cheese in a bowl.

- Top with mixed berries.

- Sprinkle ground flaxseed over the top.

- Drizzle with honey if desired.

Cooking Time: 5 minutes

Number of Servings: 1

Nutritional Information:

- Calories: 220
- Protein: 24g
- Carbohydrates: 20g
- Fiber: 5g
- Fat: 5g

Avocado and Egg Breakfast Muffins

Ingredients:

- 4 large eggs
- 1 ripe avocado, diced
- 1/4 cup diced red bell pepper
- 1/4 cup chopped spinach
- Salt and pepper to taste
- Cooking spray

Preparation:

- Preheat the oven to 350°F (175°C).

- Spray a muffin tin with cooking spray.

- In a bowl, mix the eggs until well beaten.

- Add the diced avocado, bell pepper, and spinach to the eggs.

- Turn the mixture evenly into the muffin tin.

- For 15-20 minutes, bake or until the eggs are set.

Cooking Time: 20 minutes

Number of Servings: 4 muffins

Nutritional Information (per muffin):

- Calories: 120
- Protein: 7g
- Carbohydrates: 3g
- Fiber: 2g
- Fat: 9g

Protein Smoothie

Ingredients:

- 1 scoop protein powder (whey or plant-based)
- 1 cup unsweetened almond milk
- 1/2 cup frozen berries
- 1/2 banana
- 1 tablespoon chia seeds

Preparation:

- Combine all ingredients in a blender.

- Blend until smooth.

- Pour into a glass and enjoy.

Cooking Time: 5 minutes

Number of Servings: 1

Nutritional Information:

- Calories: 250
- Protein: 20g
- Carbohydrates: 30g
- Fiber: 8g
- Fat: 7g

Oatmeal with Protein Powder

Ingredients:

- 1/2 cup rolled oats
- 1 cup water or unsweetened almond milk
- 1 scoop vanilla protein powder
- 1/4 cup fresh berries
- 1 tablespoon chopped nuts (optional)

Preparation:

- In a small pot, bring water or almond milk to a boil.

- Add the oats and reduce heat to simmer for about 5 minutes, stirring occasionally.

- Once the oats are cooked, remove from heat and stir in the protein powder.

- Top with fresh berries and chopped nuts if desired.

Cooking Time: 10 minutes

Number of Servings: 1

Nutritional Information:

- Calories: 350
- Protein: 25g
- Carbohydrates: 45g
- Fiber: 8g
- Fat: 8g

Turkey and Spinach Breakfast Roll-Ups

Ingredients:

- 2 slices turkey breast (deli-style, low sodium)
- 1/4 cup baby spinach leaves
- 1 tablespoon light cream cheese
- 1/4 avocado, sliced

Preparation:

- The turkey slices should be laid flat on a plate.

- A thin layer of light cream cheese should be spread on each slice.

- Place the spinach leaves evenly over the cream cheese.

- Add avocado slices on top.

- Roll up each turkey slice tightly and secure with a toothpick if necessary.

Cooking Time: 5 minutes

Number of Servings: 1

Nutritional Information:

- Calories: 150
- Protein: 12g
- Carbohydrates: 6g
- Fiber: 3g
- Fat: 8g

Quinoa Breakfast Bowl

Ingredients:

- 1/2 cup cooked quinoa
- 1/4 cup diced apple
- 1 tablespoon chopped walnuts
- 1/2 teaspoon cinnamon
- 1 teaspoon honey (optional)
- 1/4 cup unsweetened almond milk

Preparation:

- In a bowl, combine the cooked quinoa and diced apple.

- Sprinkle with chopped walnuts and cinnamon.

- Drizzle with honey if desired.

- Pour unsweetened almond milk over the mixture and stir to combine.

Cooking Time: 5 minutes (if quinoa is pre-cooked)

Number of Servings: 1

Nutritional Information:

- Calories: 220
- Protein: 6g
- Carbohydrates: 34g
- Fiber: 5g
- Fat: 8g

Cottage Cheese Pancakes

Ingredients:

- 1/2 cup low-fat cottage cheese
- 1/4 cup oats
- 2 egg whites
- 1/2 teaspoon vanilla extract
- Cooking spray

Preparation:

- Blend the cottage cheese, oats, egg whites, and vanilla extract in a blender until smooth.

- A non-stick skillet should be sprayed with cooking spray and heat over medium heat.

- Small amounts of the batter should be poured onto the skillet to form pancakes.

- Cook until bubbles form on the surface, then turn and cook until golden brown on both sides.

Cooking Time: 10 minutes

Number of Servings: 1 (3-4 small pancakes)

Nutritional Information:

- Calories: 200
- Protein: 20g
- Carbohydrates: 20g
- Fiber: 3g
- Fat: 4g

Smoked Salmon and Cream Cheese Roll-Ups

Ingredients:

- 2 ounces smoked salmon
- 2 tablespoons light cream cheese
- 1/4 avocado, sliced
- 1 tablespoon chopped fresh dill
- 1 teaspoon lemon juice
- Black pepper to taste

Preparation:

- Lay the smoked salmon slices flat on a plate.

- A thin layer of light cream cheese should be spread on each slice.

- Then place avocado slices on top of the cream cheese.

- Sprinkle with chopped fresh dill and drizzle with lemon juice.

- Add a dash of black pepper.

- Roll up each salmon slice tightly and secure with a toothpick if necessary.

Cooking Time: 5 minutes

Number of Servings: 1

Nutritional Information:

- Calories: 180
- Protein: 15g
- Carbohydrates: 5g
- Fiber: 3g
- Fat: 12g

Chapter Nine

Wholesome Lunch Ideas for Gastric Sleeve Patients

Chicken and Veggie Lettuce Wraps

Ingredients:

- 4 large lettuce leaves (like romaine or butter lettuce)
- 1 cup cooked, shredded chicken breast
- 1/2 cup diced cucumber
- 1/2 cup shredded carrots
- 1/4 cup chopped red bell pepper
- 1 tablespoon low-fat Greek yogurt
- 1 tablespoon lime juice
- Salt and pepper to taste

Preparation:

- In a bowl, mix the shredded chicken, diced cucumber, shredded carrots, and chopped red bell pepper.

- In a small bowl, combine the Greek yogurt and lime juice.

- Add salt and pepper to taste.

- Pour the yogurt mixture over the chicken and vegetables, and mix well.

- Using a spoon, scoop the chicken and vegetable mixture into the lettuce leaves.

- Fold the lettuce leaves around the filling to form wraps.

Cooking Time: 10 minutes

Number of Servings: 2

Nutritional Information (per serving):

- Calories: 150
- Protein: 20g
- Carbohydrates: 8g
- Fiber: 2g
- Fat: 4g

Tuna and Avocado Salad

Ingredients:

- 1 can (5 ounces) of tuna in water, drained
- 1/2 ripe avocado, diced
- 1/4 cup diced cucumber
- 1 tablespoon chopped red onion
- 1 tablespoon light mayonnaise or Greek yogurt
- 1 teaspoon lemon juice
- Salt and pepper to taste

Preparation:

- In a bowl, combine the tuna, diced avocado, diced cucumber, and chopped red onion.

- In a small bowl, mix the light mayonnaise (or Greek yogurt) and lemon juice.

- Turn the dressing over the tuna mixture and mix well.

- Season with salt and pepper to taste.

Cooking Time: 5 minutes

Number of Servings: 1

Nutritional Information:

- Calories: 220
- Protein: 25g
- Carbohydrates: 10g
- Fiber: 5g
- Fat: 10g

Quinoa and Black Bean Salad

Ingredients:

- 1/2 cup cooked quinoa
- 1/2 cup of rinsed and drained canned black beans
- 1/4 cup diced red bell pepper
- 1/4 cup diced cucumber
- 1/4 cup chopped cherry tomatoes
- 1 tablespoon chopped fresh cilantro
- 1 tablespoon lime juice
- 1 teaspoon olive oil
- Salt and pepper to taste

Preparation:

- In a large bowl, combine the cooked quinoa, black beans, diced red bell pepper, diced cucumber, chopped cherry tomatoes, and chopped cilantro.

- In a small bowl, combine the lime juice and olive oil and whisk

- Add salt and pepper to taste.

- Turn the dressing over the quinoa and vegetable mixture and toss to combine.

Cooking Time: 10 minutes (if quinoa is pre-cooked)

Number of Servings: 2

Nutritional Information (per serving):

- Calories: 250
- Protein: 8g
- Carbohydrates: 40g
- Fiber: 8g
- Fat: 6g

Turkey and Veggie Roll-Ups

Ingredients:

- 4 slices deli-style turkey breast (low sodium)

- 1/4 cup hummus
- 1/2 cucumber, cut into thin strips
- 1/2 red bell pepper, diced into thin strips
- 1/4 avocado, sliced
- Handful of baby spinach leaves

Preparation:

- Lay the turkey slices flat on a clean surface.

- Spread a thin layer of hummus on each turkey slice.

- Place cucumber strips, red bell pepper strips, avocado slices, and baby spinach leaves on top of the hummus.

- Roll up each turkey slice tightly, securing with a toothpick if necessary.

Cooking Time: 5 minutes

Number of Servings: 2

Nutritional Information (per serving):

- Calories: 180
- Protein: 18g
- Carbohydrates: 8g

- Fiber: 4g
- Fat: 9g

Shrimp and Avocado Salad

Ingredients:

- 1 cup cooked shrimp, peeled and deveined
- 1/2 avocado, diced
- 1/4 cup diced cucumber
- 1/4 cup diced red onion
- 1 tablespoon lime juice
- 1 teaspoon olive oil
- Salt and pepper to taste

Preparation:

- In a bowl, combine the cooked shrimp, diced avocado, diced cucumber, and diced red onion.

- In a small bowl, combine the lime juice and olive oil and whisk

- Add salt and pepper to taste.

- Turn the dressing over the shrimp mixture and toss to combine.

Cooking Time: 10 minutes (if shrimp is pre-cooked)

Number of Servings: 1

Nutritional Information:

- Calories: 250
- Protein: 22g
- Carbohydrates: 10g
- Fiber: 5g
- Fat: 14g

Zucchini Noodles with Pesto and Grilled Chicken

Ingredients:

- 1 medium zucchini, spiralized
- 1/2 cup cooked, diced grilled chicken breast
- 2 tablespoons pesto sauce (store-bought or homemade)
- 1 tablespoon grated Parmesan cheese (optional)
- Salt and pepper to taste

Preparation:

- In a large bowl, toss the zucchini noodles with the pesto sauce.

- Add the diced grilled chicken breast and mix well.

- Sprinkle with grated Parmesan cheese if desired.

- Season with salt and pepper to taste.

Cooking Time: 5 minutes

Number of Servings: 1

Nutritional Information:

- Calories: 300
- Protein: 28g
- Carbohydrates: 8g
- Fiber: 2g
- Fat: 18g

Egg Salad Stuffed Tomatoes

Ingredients:

- 2 large tomatoes
- 2 hard-boiled eggs, chopped

- 2 tablespoons light mayonnaise or Greek yogurt
- 1 teaspoon Dijon mustard
- 1 tablespoon chopped green onions
- Salt and pepper to taste

Preparation:

- Cut the tops off the tomatoes and scoop out the insides, leaving a hollow shell.

- In a bowl, combine the chopped hard-boiled eggs, light mayonnaise (or Greek yogurt), Dijon mustard, and chopped green onions.

- Season with salt and pepper to taste.

- Spoon the egg salad mixture into the hollowed-out tomatoes.

Cooking Time: 10 minutes

Number of Servings: 2

Nutritional Information (per serving):

- Calories: 200
- Protein: 12g
- Carbohydrates: 10g

- Fiber: 3g
- Fat: 14g

Greek Yogurt Chicken Salad

Ingredients:

- 1 cup cooked, shredded chicken breast
- 1/4 cup plain Greek yogurt
- 1 tablespoon lemon juice
- 1/4 cup diced celery
- 1/4 cup diced apple
- 1 tablespoon chopped fresh parsley
- Salt and pepper to taste

Preparation:

- In a bowl, combine the shredded chicken, Greek yogurt, and lemon juice.

- Add the diced celery, diced apple, and chopped parsley.

- Mix well.

- Season with salt and pepper to taste.

- Serve chilled.

Cooking Time: 10 minutes

Number of Servings: 1

Nutritional Information:

- Calories: 250
- Protein: 30g
- Carbohydrates: 12g
- Fiber: 3g
- Fat: 8g

Spaghetti Squash with Turkey Bolognese

Ingredients:

- 1 small spaghetti squash
- 1 cup ground turkey (lean)
- 1/2 cup marinara sauce (low-sodium)
- 1/4 cup diced onion
- 1 clove garlic, minced
- 1 tablespoon olive oil
- 1 teaspoon Italian seasoning
- Salt and pepper to taste
- Fresh basil for garnish (optional)

Preparation:

- Preheat the oven to 400°F (200°C).

- The spaghetti squash should be cut into half lengthwise and remove the seeds.

- Drizzle the cut sides with olive oil and place face down on a baking sheet.

- Roast in the oven for 30-40 minutes, or until the flesh is tender and can be easily shredded with a fork.

- While the squash is roasting, heat a skillet over medium heat and add the olive oil.

- Sauté the diced onion and minced garlic until fragrant and translucent, about 3-4 minutes.

- Add the ground turkey to the skillet, cook until browned, breaking it apart with a spoon.

- Stir in the marinara sauce and Italian seasoning.

- For 10 minutes, simmer to allow the flavors to combine.

- Add salt and pepper to taste.

- Once the spaghetti squash is cooked, use a fork to scrape out the flesh into strands and place it in a bowl.

- Top the spaghetti squash with the turkey Bolognese sauce.

- Garnish with fresh basil if desired.

Cooking Time: 50 minutes

Number of Servings: 2

Nutritional Information (per serving):

- Calories: 300
- Protein: 25g
- Carbohydrates: 20g
- Fiber: 4g
- Fat: 12g

Lentil and Vegetable Soup

Ingredients:

- 1/2 cup dried lentils, rinsed
- 1 small carrot, diced
- 1 small celery stalk, diced

- 1/2 onion, diced
- 1 small zucchini, diced
- 2 cups low-sodium vegetable broth
- 1 cup water
- 1 clove garlic, minced
- 1 teaspoon olive oil
- 1/2 teaspoon cumin
- 1/2 teaspoon paprika
- Salt and pepper to taste
- Fresh parsley for garnish (optional)

Preparation:

- In a large pot, heat the olive oil over medium heat.

- Combine the diced onion, carrot, celery, and minced garlic.

- For about 5 minutes, sauté until the vegetables are soft.

- Add the cumin and paprika, and cook for another minute while stirring.

- Combine the lentils, vegetable broth, and water to the pot.

- Bring to a boil.

- Reduce the heat to low, cover, and simmer for about 25-30 minutes, or until the lentils are tender.

- Add the diced zucchini and continue to cook for another 5-10 minutes, until the zucchini is tender.

- Season with salt and pepper to taste.

- If desired, before serving, garnish with fresh parsley.

Cooking Time: 45 minutes

Number of Servings: 2

Nutritional Information (per serving):

- Calories: 220
- Protein: 12g
- Carbohydrates: 35g
- Fiber: 12g
- Fat: 4g

Chapter Ten

Nourishing Dinners for Gastric Sleeve Patients

Baked Salmon with Asparagus

Ingredients:

- 2 salmon fillets (4 ounces each)
- 1 bunch asparagus, trimmed
- 1 tablespoon olive oil
- 1 lemon, sliced
- 1 teaspoon garlic powder
- 1 teaspoon dried dill
- Salt and pepper to taste

Preparation:

- Preheat the oven to 400°F (200°C).

- A baking sheet should be lined with parchment paper or foil.

- The salmon fillets and asparagus should be placed on the baking sheet.

- Drizzle olive oil on the salmon and asparagus.

- Sprinkle garlic powder, dried dill, salt, and pepper over the salmon and asparagus.

- On top of the salmon fillets, arrange lemon slices

- For 15-20 minutes, bake or until the salmon is thoroughly cooked and flakes easily with a fork, and the asparagus is soft.

Cooking Time: 25 minutes

Number of Servings: 2

Nutritional Information (per serving):

- Calories: 300
- Protein: 30g
- Carbohydrates: 8g
- Fiber: 4g
- Fat: 16g

Turkey Meatballs with Zoodles

Ingredients:

- 1/2 pound ground turkey (lean)
- 1/4 cup grated Parmesan cheese
- 1/4 cup breadcrumbs (optional)
- 1 egg, beaten
- 1 teaspoon garlic powder
- 1 teaspoon onion powder
- 1 teaspoon Italian seasoning
- 2 medium zucchinis, spiralized
- 1 cup marinara sauce (low-sodium)
- 1 tablespoon olive oil
- Salt and pepper to taste

Preparation:

- Preheat the oven to 375°F (190°C).

- In a large bowl, add the ground turkey, Parmesan cheese, breadcrumbs (if using), egg, garlic powder, onion powder, Italian seasoning, salt, and pepper.

- Mould the mixture into small meatballs and place them on a baking sheet lined with parchment paper.

- Bake for 20-25 minutes, or until the meatballs are cooked through and golden brown.

- The olive oil should be heated in a large skillet over medium heat while the meatballs are baking.

- Add the spiralized zucchini (zoodles) to the skillet and sauté for 2-3 minutes, until slightly tender.

- The marinara sauce should be added to the skillet and heat through.

- Serve the meatballs over the zoodles.

Cooking Time: 30 minutes

Number of Servings: 2

Nutritional Information (per serving):

- Calories: 350
- Protein: 28g
- Carbohydrates: 18g
- Fiber: 5g
- Fat: 18g

Stuffed Bell Peppers

Ingredients:

- 2 large bell peppers, halved and seeds removed
- 1/2 pound ground chicken or turkey
- 1/2 cup cooked quinoa
- 1/2 cup diced tomatoes
- 1/4 cup diced onion
- 1 clove garlic, minced
- 1 teaspoon cumin
- 1 teaspoon chili powder
- 1 tablespoon olive oil
- 1/4 cup shredded low-fat cheese (optional)
- Salt and pepper to taste

Preparation:

- Preheat the oven to 375°F (190°C).

- The olive oil should be heated in a large skillet over medium heat.

- Add the diced onion and minced garlic to the skillet and sauté until translucent, about 3-4 minutes.

- Add the ground chicken or turkey to the skillet and cook until browned, breaking it apart with a spoon.

- Stir in the diced tomatoes, cooked quinoa, cumin, chili powder, salt, and pepper.

- Cook for another 2-3 minutes until well combined and heated through.

- Place the bell pepper halves in a baking dish and stuff them with the meat and quinoa mixture.

- Top with shredded cheese if desired.

- Cover the stuffed bell pepper with foil and bake for 25-30 minutes, or until the peppers are soft.

Cooking Time: 40 minutes

Number of Servings: 2

Nutritional Information (per serving):

- Calories: 300
- Protein: 25g
- Carbohydrates: 25g

- Fiber: 6g
- Fat: 12g

Cauliflower Fried Rice with Chicken

Ingredients:

- 1 medium head of cauliflower, grated or processed into rice-sized pieces
- 1 cup cooked, diced chicken breast
- 1/2 cup frozen peas and carrots mix
- 1/4 cup diced onion
- 2 cloves garlic, minced
- 2 eggs, beaten
- 2 tablespoons low-sodium soy sauce
- 1 tablespoon sesame oil
- 1 tablespoon olive oil
- Salt and pepper to taste
- Green onions for garnish (optional)

Preparation:

- The olive oil should be heated in a large skillet over medium heat.

- Add the diced onion and garlic and sauté until fragrant and translucent, about 3-4 minutes.

- Add the frozen peas and carrots and cook for another 2-3 minutes until thawed and slightly tender.

- Pack the vegetables to one side of the skillet and pour the beaten eggs into the empty side.

- Scramble the eggs until cooked, then mix with the vegetables.

- Add the grated cauliflower to the skillet and cook for 5-7 minutes, stirring occasionally, until the cauliflower is tender.

- Stir in the cooked chicken, low-sodium soy sauce, and sesame oil.

- For an additional 2-3 minutes, cook until everything is well combined and thoroughly heated.

- Season with salt and pepper to taste.

- Garnish with green onions if desired.

Cooking Time: 20 minutes

Number of Servings: 2

Nutritional Information (per serving):

- Calories: 280
- Protein: 25g
- Carbohydrates: 12g
- Fiber: 5g
- Fat: 14g

Baked Cod with Vegetables

Ingredients:

- 2 cod fillets (4 ounces each)
- 1 cup cherry tomatoes, halved
- 1 small zucchini, sliced
- 1/2 red onion, sliced
- 2 cloves garlic, minced
- 1 tablespoon olive oil
- 1 teaspoon dried oregano
- 1 lemon, sliced
- Salt and pepper to taste
- Fresh parsley for garnish (optional)

Preparation:

- Preheat the oven to 375°F (190°C).

- In a large baking dish, combine the cherry tomatoes, sliced zucchini, sliced red onion, minced garlic, olive oil, dried oregano, salt, and pepper.

- Toss to coat the vegetables evenly.

- Place the cod fillets on top of the vegetables and season with salt and pepper.

- On top of the cod fillets, arrange lemon slices

- Cover the baking dish with foil and bake for 20-25 minutes, or until the cod is cooked through and flakes easily with a fork.

- If desired, before serving, garnish with fresh parsley.

Cooking Time: 30 minutes

Number of Servings: 2

Nutritional Information (per serving):

- Calories: 250
- Protein: 25g
- Carbohydrates: 14g

- Fiber: 4g
- Fat: 10g

Stuffed Portobello Mushrooms

Ingredients:

- 4 large portobello mushrooms, stems removed
- 1 cup fresh spinach, chopped
- 1/2 cup ricotta cheese (low-fat)
- 1/4 cup grated Parmesan cheese
- 1 clove garlic, minced
- 1 tablespoon olive oil
- 1/2 teaspoon dried basil
- 1/2 teaspoon dried oregano
- Salt and pepper to taste

Preparation:

- Preheat the oven to 375°F (190°C).

- Brush the portobello mushrooms with olive oil and place them on a baking sheet.

- In a bowl, combine the chopped spinach, ricotta cheese, Parmesan cheese, minced garlic, dried basil, dried oregano, salt, and pepper.

- The mushroom caps should be stuffed with the spinach and cheese mixture.

- Bake for 20-25 minutes, or until the mushrooms are tender and the filling is heated through.

Cooking Time: 30 minutes

Number of Servings: 2

Nutritional Information (per serving):

- Calories: 200
- Protein: 14g
- Carbohydrates: 10g
- Fiber: 3g
- Fat: 13g

Baked Chicken Parmesan

Ingredients:

- 2 boneless, skinless chicken breasts (4 ounces per one)
- 1/2 cup marinara sauce (low-sodium)
- 1/4 cup grated Parmesan cheese

- 1/4 cup mozzarella cheese (low-fat), shredded
- 1/4 cup whole wheat breadcrumbs
- 1 tablespoon olive oil
- 1 teaspoon Italian seasoning
- Salt and pepper to taste

Preparation:

- Preheat the oven to 375°F (190°C).

- The chicken breasts should be pounded to a uniform thickness.

- In a bowl, mix the breadcrumbs, Parmesan cheese, Italian seasoning, salt, and pepper.

- Dip the chicken breasts in olive oil and then coat with the breadcrumb mixture.

- The chicken should be placed on a baking sheet and bake for 20-25 minutes, or until the chicken is thoroughly cooked.

- Each chicken breast should be topped with marinara sauce and shredded mozzarella cheese.

- Return the topped chicken breast to the oven for another 5 minutes, or until the cheese is melted and bubbly.

Cooking Time: 30 minutes

Number of Servings: 2

Nutritional Information (per serving):

- Calories: 320
- Protein: 30g
- Carbohydrates: 12g
- Fiber: 2g
- Fat: 16g

Shrimp Stir-Fry with Broccoli

Ingredients:

- 1/2 pound shrimp, peeled and deveined
- 2 cups broccoli florets
- 1/2 bell pepper, sliced
- 1/2 onion, sliced
- 2 cloves garlic, minced
- 2 tablespoons low-sodium soy sauce
- 1 tablespoon olive oil
- 1 teaspoon sesame oil
- 1 teaspoon grated ginger

- Salt and pepper to taste

Preparation:

- The olive oil should be heated in a large skillet over medium-high heat.

- Add the minced garlic and grated ginger and sauté for 1-2 minutes.

- Add the broccoli florets, sliced bell pepper, and sliced onion to the skillet.

- For 5-7 minutes, cook until the vegetables are tender-crisp.

- Add the shrimp to the skillet and cook for another 3-4 minutes, until the shrimp are pink and opaque.

- Add the low-sodium soy sauce and sesame oil and stir.

- For another minute, cook until everything is well combined.

- To taste, season with salt and pepper.

Cooking Time: 20 minutes

Number of Servings: 2

Nutritional Information (per serving):

- Calories: 250
- Protein: 25g
- Carbohydrates: 14g
- Fiber: 5g
- Fat: 10g

Turkey and Sweet Potato Skillet

Ingredients:

- 1/2 pound ground turkey (lean)
- 1 medium sweet potato, peeled and diced
- 1/2 red bell pepper, diced
- 1/2 onion, diced
- 2 cloves garlic, minced
- 1 tablespoon olive oil
- 1 teaspoon smoked paprika
- 1/2 teaspoon cumin
- Salt and pepper to taste
- Fresh cilantro for garnish (optional)

Preparation:

- The olive oil should be heated in a large skillet over medium heat.

- Add the diced onion and minced garlic and sauté until translucent, about 3-4 minutes.

- Add the ground turkey to the skillet and cook until browned, while breaking it apart with a spoon.

- Stir in the diced sweet potato, diced red bell pepper, smoked paprika, cumin, salt, and pepper.

- Cover and cook for 10-15 minutes, stirring occasionally, until the sweet potato is tender.

- If desired, before serving, garnish with fresh cilantro.

Cooking Time: 25 minutes

Number of Servings: 2

Nutritional Information (per serving):

- Calories: 320

- Protein: 25g
- Carbohydrates: 30g
- Fiber: 5g
- Fat: 12g

Tilapia with Lemon and Capers

Ingredients:

- 2 tilapia fillets (4 ounces each)
- 1 tablespoon olive oil
- 1 lemon, thinly sliced
- 1 tablespoon capers, drained
- 1/2 teaspoon garlic powder
- Salt and pepper to taste
- Fresh parsley for garnish (optional)

Preparation:

- Preheat the oven to 375°F (190°C).

- Place the tilapia fillets on a baking sheet lined with parchment paper.

- Drizzle the olive oil over the fillets and season with garlic powder, salt, and pepper.

- Arrange the lemon slices on top of the fillets and sprinkle with capers.

- For 15-20 minutes, bake or until the tilapia is thoroughly cooked and flakes easily with a fork.

- If desired, before serving, garnish with fresh parsley.

Cooking Time: 20 minutes

Number of Servings: 2

Nutritional Information (per serving):

- Calories: 220
- Protein: 22g
- Carbohydrates: 6g
- Fiber: 2g
- Fat: 12g

Chapter Eleven

Gastric Sleeve-Friendly Snack Options

Greek Yogurt with Berries

Ingredients:

- 1 cup plain Greek yogurt (low-fat)
- 1/2 cup mixed berries (strawberries, blueberries, raspberries)
- 1 teaspoon honey (optional)
- 1 tablespoon chopped nuts (like almonds, walnuts, or pecans)

Preparation:

- Spoon the Greek yogurt into a bowl.

- Top with mixed berries.

- Drizzle with honey if desired.

- Sprinkle with chopped nuts.

Cooking Time: 5 minutes

Number of Servings: 1

Nutritional Information (per serving):

- Calories: 200
- Protein: 18g
- Carbohydrates: 20g
- Fiber: 4g
- Fat: 7g

Hummus and Veggie Sticks

Ingredients:

- 1/2 cup hummus
- 1 carrot, cut into sticks
- 1 cucumber, cut into sticks
- 1 bell pepper, cut into sticks
- 1 celery stalk, cut into sticks

Preparation:

- Arrange the vegetable sticks on a plate.

- Serve with hummus for dipping.

Cooking Time: 5 minutes

Number of Servings: 2

Nutritional Information (per serving):

- Calories: 150
- Protein: 5g
- Carbohydrates: 20g
- Fiber: 6g
- Fat: 6g

Cottage Cheese with Pineapple

Ingredients:

- 1 cup cottage cheese (low-fat)
- 1/2 cup fresh or canned pineapple chunks in juice, drained
- 1 tablespoon chia seeds (optional)

Preparation:

- Spoon the cottage cheese into a bowl.

- Top with pineapple chunks.

- Sprinkle with chia seeds if desired.

Cooking Time: 5 minutes

Number of Servings: 1

Nutritional Information (per serving):

- Calories: 180
- Protein: 20g
- Carbohydrates: 18g
- Fiber: 3g
- Fat: 4g

Apple Slices with Peanut Butter

Ingredients:

- 1 medium apple, sliced
- 2 tablespoons natural, no added sugar peanut butter

Preparation:

- Slice the apple into thin wedges.

- Serve with peanut butter for dipping.

Cooking Time: 5 minutes

Number of Servings: 1

Nutritional Information (per serving):

- Calories: 200
- Protein: 4g
- Carbohydrates: 28g
- Fiber: 6g
- Fat: 9g

Turkey and Cheese Roll-Ups

Ingredients:

- 4 slices deli turkey breast (low sodium)
- 2 slices low-fat cheese (such as Swiss or cheddar)
- 1/2 avocado, sliced
- 1 teaspoon Dijon mustard (optional)

Preparation:

- Lay the turkey slices flat on a clean surface.

- Place a cheese slice and avocado slice on each turkey slice.

- Add a small amount of Dijon mustard if desired.

- Roll up each turkey slice tightly.

Cooking Time: 5 minutes

Number of Servings: 2

Nutritional Information (per serving):

- Calories: 180
- Protein: 16g
- Carbohydrates: 6g
- Fiber: 3g
- Fat: 10g

Cottage Cheese and Tomato Slices

Ingredients:

- 1/2 cup cottage cheese (low-fat)
- 1 medium tomato, sliced
- Fresh basil leaves, chopped (optional)
- Balsamic glaze (optional)

Preparation:

- Place cottage cheese in a bowl.

- Arrange tomato slices on top.

- Garnish with chopped basil leaves.

- Drizzle with balsamic glaze if desired.

Number of Servings: 1

Nutritional Information (per serving):

- Calories: 150
- Protein: 15g
- Carbohydrates: 12g
- Fiber: 3g
- Fat: 5g

Almond Butter and Banana Slices on Rice Cakes

Ingredients:

- 2 rice cakes (unsalted)
- 2 tablespoons almond butter (unsweetened)
- 1 small banana, sliced

Preparation:

- Spread almond butter evenly on rice cakes.

- Top with banana slices.

Number of Servings: 1

Nutritional Information (per serving):

- Calories: 280
- Protein: 7g
- Carbohydrates: 34g
- Fiber: 5g
- Fat: 14g

Hard-Boiled Eggs and Baby Carrots

Ingredients:

- 2 hard-boiled eggs
- 1 cup baby carrots

Preparation:

- Peel hard-boiled eggs.

- Serve with baby carrots.

Number of Servings: 1

Nutritional Information (per serving):

- Calories: 200

- Protein: 12g
- Carbohydrates: 14g
- Fiber: 4g
- Fat: 10g

Turkey and Cheese Roll-Ups with Cucumber Slices

Ingredients:

- 4 slices deli turkey breast (low sodium)
- 2 slices low-fat cheese
- 1/2 cucumber, sliced

Preparation:

- Lay turkey slices flat.

- Place cheese slices on each.

- Roll up and serve with cucumber slices.

Number of Servings: 1

Nutritional Information (per serving):

- Calories: 180
- Protein: 16g
- Carbohydrates: 6g

- Fiber: 2g
- Fat: 10g

Greek Yogurt with Almonds and Honey

Ingredients:

- 1/2 cup plain Greek yogurt (low-fat)
- 1 tablespoon almonds, chopped
- 1 teaspoon honey

Preparation:

- Place Greek yogurt in a bowl.

- Sprinkle chopped almonds on top.

- Drizzle with honey.

Number of Servings: 1

Nutritional Information (per serving):

- Calories: 200
- Protein: 18g
- Carbohydrates: 16g
- Fiber: 2g
- Fat: 9g

Indulgent Desserts for Gastric Sleeve Patients

Greek Yogurt Parfait

Ingredients:

- 1/2 cup plain Greek yogurt (low-fat)
- 1/4 cup mixed berries (strawberries, blueberries, raspberries)
- 1 tablespoon chopped nuts (almonds, walnuts)
- 1 teaspoon honey (optional)

Preparation:

- **Spoon Greek yogurt** into a serving glass.

- Layer with mixed berries and chopped nuts.

- Drizzle with honey if desired.

Number of Servings: 1

Nutritional Information (per serving):

- Calories: 180
- Protein: 15g
- Carbohydrates: 15g
- Fiber: 3g

- Fat: 8g

Chocolate Protein Pudding

Ingredients:

- 1 scoop chocolate protein powder
- 1/2 cup unsweetened almond milk
- 1 tablespoon unsweetened cocoa powder
- 1 tablespoon chia seeds
- Stevia or monk fruit sweetener to taste

Preparation:

- In a bowl, mix together chocolate protein powder, unsweetened cocoa powder, chia seeds, and sweetener.

- Slowly stir in almond milk until mixture thickens.

- For at least 30 minutes, chill in the refrigerator before serving.

Number of Servings: 1

Nutritional Information (per serving):

- Calories: 200

- Protein: 25g
- Carbohydrates: 10g
- Fiber: 5g
- Fat: 6g

Frozen Yogurt Bark

Ingredients:

- 1 cup plain Greek yogurt (low-fat)
- 1 tablespoon honey or maple syrup
- 1/4 cup mixed berries (strawberries, blueberries)
- 2 tablespoons chopped nuts (almonds, walnuts)

Preparation:

- In a bowl, add together Greek yogurt and honey or maple syrup and mix.

- Line a baking sheet with parchment paper.

- Spread yogurt mixture evenly onto the parchment paper.

- Sprinkle mixed berries and chopped nuts over the yogurt.

- Freeze for 2-3 hours until firm.

- Break into pieces and serve.

Number of Servings: 4

Nutritional Information (per serving):

- Calories: 70
- Protein: 5g
- Carbohydrates: 7g
- Fiber: 1g
- Fat: 3g

Baked Apples with Cinnamon

Ingredients:

- 2 apples, cored and halved
- 1 tablespoon lemon juice
- 1 teaspoon cinnamon
- 1 tablespoon chopped nuts (almonds, walnuts)
- 1 tablespoon raisins (optional)
- Stevia or monk fruit sweetener to taste

Preparation:

- Preheat oven to 375°F (190°C).

- Place apple halves in a baking dish.

- Drizzle lemon juice over apples.

- Sprinkle with cinnamon, chopped nuts, and raisins.

- For 20-25 minutes, bake until the apples are soft.

- Serve warm.

Number of Servings: 2

Nutritional Information (per serving):

- Calories: 100
- Protein: 1g
- Carbohydrates: 20g
- Fiber: 5g
- Fat: 3g

Chia Seed Pudding with Berries

Ingredients:

- 2 tablespoons chia seeds
- 1/2 cup unsweetened almond milk

- 1/4 teaspoon vanilla extract
- Stevia or monk fruit sweetener to taste
- 1/4 cup mixed berries (strawberries, blueberries)

Preparation:

- In a bowl, mix together chia seeds, almond milk, vanilla extract, and sweetener.

- Refrigerate for at least 2 hours or overnight until mixture thickens.

- Serve topped with mixed berries.

Number of Servings: 1

Nutritional Information (per serving):

- Calories: 120
- Protein: 4g
- Carbohydrates: 12g
- Fiber: 8g
- Fat: 7g

Protein Peanut Butter Cups

Ingredients:

- 2 tablespoons natural, no added sugar peanut butter
- 1 scoop chocolate protein powder
- 2 tablespoons unsweetened almond milk

Preparation:

- In a bowl, mix together peanut butter, chocolate protein powder, and almond milk until well combined.

- Spoon mixture into mini muffin liners or silicone molds.

- Freeze for 30 minutes until firm.

- Remove from molds and enjoy.

Number of Servings: 2

Nutritional Information (per serving):

- Calories: 200
- Protein: 20g
- Carbohydrates: 8g

- Fiber: 3g
- Fat: 10g

Banana "Nice Cream"

Ingredients:

- 1 ripe banana, sliced and frozen
- 1 tablespoon unsweetened cocoa powder
- 1 tablespoon almond milk (optional)

Preparation:

- The frozen banana slices should be placed in a blender or food processor.

- Add cocoa powder and almond milk.

- Blend until smooth and creamy.

- Serve immediately.

Number of Servings: 1

Nutritional Information (per serving):

- Calories: 150
- Protein: 2g
- Carbohydrates: 35g

- Fiber: 5g
- Fat: 1g

Protein Pancakes

Ingredients:

- 1 scoop vanilla protein powder
- 1/4 cup egg whites
- 1/4 cup oats
- 1/4 teaspoon baking powder
- Stevia or monk fruit sweetener to taste
- 1/4 cup unsweetened almond milk

Preparation:

- In a blender, combine protein powder, egg whites, oats, baking powder, sweetener, and almond milk.

- Blend until smooth.

- Heat a non-stick skillet over medium heat.

- Pour batter onto the skillet to form pancakes.

- The pancakes should be cooked until bubbles form on the surface, then flip and cook until golden brown.

- Serve with fresh berries or sugar-free syrup.

Number of Servings: 1 (2 small pancakes)

Nutritional Information (per serving):

- Calories: 250
- Protein: 30g
- Carbohydrates: 20g
- Fiber: 4g
- Fat: 6g

Coconut Chia Seed Pudding

Ingredients:

- 2 tablespoons chia seeds
- 1/2 cup unsweetened coconut milk
- 1/4 teaspoon vanilla extract
- Stevia or monk fruit sweetener to taste
- 1 tablespoon shredded coconut (unsweetened)

Preparation:

- In a bowl, mix together chia seeds, coconut milk, vanilla extract, and sweetener.

- Refrigerate for at least 2 hours or overnight until mixture thickens.

- Serve topped with shredded coconut.

Number of Servings: 1

Nutritional Information (per serving):

- Calories: 200
- Protein: 4g
- Carbohydrates: 14g
- Fiber: 10g
- Fat: 15g

Baked Pear with Cinnamon

Ingredients:

- 1 ripe pear, halved and cored
- 1 teaspoon honey (optional)
- 1/4 teaspoon cinnamon

Preparation:

- Preheat oven to 375°F (190°C).

- Pear halves, cut side up, should be placed on a baking sheet.

- Drizzle with honey and sprinkle with cinnamon.

- Bake for 20-25 minutes until pear is tender.

- Serve warm.

Number of Servings: 1

Nutritional Information (per serving):

- Calories: 100
- Protein: 1g
- Carbohydrates: 25g
- Fiber: 5g
- Fat: 0g

Chapter Twelve

A 4-week Bariatric Meal Plan

Adhering to a strict meal plan is crucial after weight reduction surgery in order to meet nutritional needs and successfully lose weight over the long run.

Meal planning for bariatric patients should aim to limit portions, minimize calories, supply enough protein, and avoid dumping syndrome. In order to maintain muscle mass as the body loses weight, patients require 70–90g of protein each day. Consistent weight loss is facilitated by consuming approximately 1200 calories each day. Frequent, small meals facilitate better digestion and help avoid overindulging. Foods low in fat and sugar have a lower chance of causing dumping syndrome, this occurs when food passes through the small intestine too quickly after leaving the stomach.

This meal plan lasts for 28 days and is intended for bariatric patients who have previously completed the first phases of the diet following surgery, which are clear liquids, pureed foods, soft foods, and solid foods. At this stage, the patient can adhere to a post-bariatric diet plan that is balanced and includes a range of foods. This meal plan aims to support optimal health and successful weight loss following gastric bypass or gastric sleeve surgery.

Week 1

Day 1:

- **Breakfast:** Protein smoothie (1 scoop protein powder, 1/2 banana, 1 cup unsweetened almond milk, handful of spinach)

- **Lunch:** Turkey and vegetable puree (1/2 cup cooked turkey breast, 1/2 cup mixed cooked vegetables, pureed with 1/4 cup low-sodium chicken broth)

- **Dinner:** Baked salmon with steamed broccoli (3 oz baked salmon seasoned with herbs and lemon juice, served with 1 cup steamed broccoli)

- **Snack:** Greek yogurt with chia seeds sprinkle over it

Day 2:

- **Breakfast:** Greek yogurt parfait (1/2 cup Greek yogurt, 1/4 cup berries, 1 tablespoon chopped nuts)

- **Lunch:** Creamy cauliflower mash (1 cup cooked cauliflower pureed with 1/4 cup unsweetened almond milk and 1 tablespoon low-fat cream cheese)

- **Dinner:** Grilled chicken breast with mashed sweet potatoes (3 oz grilled chicken breast with 1/2 cup mashed sweet potatoes)

- **Snack:** Sugar-free gelatin

Day 3:

- **Breakfast:** Vanilla protein oatmeal (1/2 cup cooked oats mixed with 1 scoop vanilla protein powder, topped with cinnamon and sliced strawberries)

- **Lunch:** Creamy spinach and ricotta pasta (1 cup cooked pasta pureed with 1 cup cooked spinach, 1/2 cup unsweetened almond milk, and 1/4 cup ricotta cheese)

- **Dinner:** Turkey meatballs with marinara sauce and zucchini noodles (3 turkey meatballs served with 1/2 cup marinara sauce and 1 cup zucchini noodles)

- **Snack:** Protein peanut butter cups (homemade)

Day 4:

- **Breakfast:** Scrambled eggs with avocado (2 scrambled eggs topped with mashed avocado)

- **Lunch:** Creamy carrot soup (1 cup cooked carrots pureed with 1 cup vegetable broth, 1/4 cup unsweetened almond milk, and spices)

- **Dinner:** Beef stir-fry with mixed vegetables (3 oz lean beef stir-fried with assorted vegetables, served with cauliflower rice)

- **Snack:** Cottage cheese with sliced cucumbers

Day 5:

- **Breakfast:** Banana coconut smoothie (1 ripe banana, 1/2 cup coconut milk, 1/2 cup unsweetened almond milk, and ice cubes)

- **Lunch:** Creamy lentil soup (1/2 cup cooked lentils pureed with 1 cup vegetable broth, 1/4 cup unsweetened almond milk, and spices)

- **Dinner:** Grilled shrimp skewers with quinoa salad (3 oz grilled shrimp skewers served with 1/2 cup quinoa salad with mixed vegetables)

- **Snack:** Sugar-free yogurt with a drizzle of honey

Day 6:

- **Breakfast:** Protein pancakes (2 pancakes made with protein powder, egg whites, and oats, served with sugar-free syrup)

- **Lunch:** Creamy mushroom puree (1 cup cooked mushrooms pureed with 1/2 cup vegetable broth, 1/4 cup unsweetened almond milk, and cream cheese)

- **Dinner:** Lemon herb baked chicken with mashed cauliflower (3 oz baked chicken breast seasoned with lemon and herbs, served with 1 cup mashed cauliflower)

- **Snack:** Chocolate avocado pudding (homemade)

Day 7:

- **Breakfast:** Blueberry protein smoothie (1 scoop protein powder, 1/2 cup blueberries, 1 cup unsweetened almond milk, and spinach)

- **Lunch:** Creamy pumpkin soup (1 cup canned pumpkin puree blended with 1 cup vegetable broth, 1/4 cup unsweetened almond milk, and spices)

- **Dinner:** Beef and vegetable stir-fry with brown rice (3 oz lean beef stir-fried with mixed vegetables, served with 1/2 cup cooked brown rice)

- **Snack:** Greek yogurt with sliced almonds

Week 2

Day 1:

- **Breakfast:** Protein oatmeal (1/2 cup cooked oats mixed with 1 scoop protein powder, topped with sliced bananas)

- **Lunch:** Creamy broccoli soup (1 cup cooked broccoli pureed with 1 cup vegetable broth, 1/4 cup unsweetened almond milk, and spices)

- **Dinner:** Baked cod with roasted asparagus (3 oz baked cod seasoned with herbs, served with 1 cup roasted asparagus)

- **Snack:** Cottage cheese with pineapple chunks

Day 2:

- **Breakfast:** Spinach and feta omelet (2 eggs scrambled with spinach and feta cheese)

- **Lunch:** Creamy chicken and potato puree (1/2 cup cooked chicken breast pureed with 1/2 cup cooked potato, 1/4 cup low-sodium chicken broth, and 1/4 cup unsweetened almond milk)

- **Dinner:** Turkey chili (3 oz ground turkey cooked with diced tomatoes, kidney beans, chili powder, and onions)

- **Snack:** Protein shake (1 scoop protein powder mixed with water or unsweetened almond milk)

Day 3:

- **Breakfast:** Greek yogurt with sliced peaches and almonds

- **Lunch:** Creamy cauliflower and leek soup (1 cup cooked cauliflower pureed with 1/2 cup cooked leeks, 1 cup vegetable broth, 1/4 cup unsweetened almond milk, and spices)

- **Dinner:** Grilled steak with mashed butternut squash (3 oz grilled steak served with 1/2 cup mashed butternut squash)

- **Snack:** Sugar-free gelatin with whipped cream

Day 4:

- **Breakfast:** Protein pancakes topped with mixed berries

- **Lunch:** Creamy mushroom risotto (1/2 cup cooked mushrooms pureed with 1/2 cup cooked brown rice, 1/4 cup unsweetened almond milk, and grated Parmesan cheese)

- **Dinner:** Lemon herb roasted chicken with steamed green beans (3 oz roasted chicken seasoned with lemon and herbs, served with 1 cup steamed green beans)

- **Snack:** Carrot and cucumber sticks with hummus

Day 5:

- **Breakfast:** Blueberry protein smoothie (1 scoop protein powder, 1/2 cup blueberries, 1/2 banana, 1 cup unsweetened almond milk)

- **Lunch:** Creamy spinach and ricotta soup (1 cup cooked spinach pureed with 1/4 cup ricotta cheese, 1 cup vegetable broth, and 1/4 cup unsweetened almond milk)

- **Dinner:** Shrimp and vegetable stir-fry with cauliflower rice (3 oz shrimp stir-fried with mixed vegetables, served with 1 cup cauliflower rice)

- **Snack:** Sugar-free yogurt with mixed nuts

Day 6:

- **Breakfast:** Vanilla protein smoothie bowl (1 scoop protein powder blended with frozen mixed berries and topped with sliced almonds)

- **Lunch:** Creamy pumpkin and ginger soup (1 cup canned pumpkin puree blended with 1/2 teaspoon ground ginger, 1 cup vegetable broth, and 1/4 cup unsweetened almond milk)

- **Dinner:** Baked tilapia with sautéed spinach (3 oz baked tilapia seasoned with lemon and herbs, served with 1 cup sautéed spinach)

- **Snack:** Protein peanut butter balls (homemade)

Day 7:

- **Breakfast:** Scrambled eggs with salsa and avocado

- **Lunch:** Creamy lentil and vegetable soup (1/2 cup cooked lentils pureed with mixed cooked vegetables, 1 cup vegetable broth, and 1/4 cup unsweetened almond milk)

- **Dinner:** Grilled chicken Caesar salad (3 oz grilled chicken breast served on a bed of romaine lettuce with Caesar dressing)

- **Snack:** Sugar-free gelatin with whipped cream

Week 3

Day 1:

- **Breakfast:** Protein smoothie made with 1 scoop of protein powder, 1/2 cup of mixed berries, and 1/2 cup of unsweetened almond milk.

- **Lunch:** Pureed chicken and vegetable soup made with cooked chicken breast, mixed vegetables, and low-sodium chicken broth.

- **Dinner:** Steamed broccoli with baked salmon fillet and quinoa.

- **Snack:** Cottage cheese with sliced peaches.

Day 2:

- **Breakfast:** Greek yogurt parfait with 1/2 cup of Greek yogurt, 1/4 cup of granola, and a handful of sliced strawberries.

- **Lunch:** Pureed lentil soup made with cooked lentils, diced tomatoes, onions, and vegetable broth.

- **Dinner:** Grilled chicken breast with mashed sweet potatoes and sautéed spinach.

- **Snack:** Sugar-free gelatin with whipped cream.

Day 3:

- **Breakfast:** Diced bell peppers and onions with scrambled eggs.

- **Lunch:** Creamy cauliflower and cheese soup made with pureed cauliflower, low-fat cheese, and vegetable broth.

- **Dinner:** Zucchini noodles served with turkey meatballs and marinara sauce.

- **Snack:** Protein shake made with 1 scoop of protein powder and 1/2 cup of unsweetened almond milk.

Day 4:

- **Breakfast:** Protein pancakes topped with sliced bananas and a drizzle of sugar-free syrup.

- **Lunch:** Pureed butternut squash soup made with roasted butternut squash, vegetable broth, and a splash of coconut milk.

- **Dinner:** Baked cod fillet with roasted Brussels sprouts and quinoa.

- **Snack:** Celery sticks with almond butter.

Day 5:

- **Breakfast:** Spinach and feta cheese omelette made with 2 eggs and a handful of spinach.

- **Lunch:** Creamy mushroom and thyme soup made with pureed mushrooms, thyme, low-sodium chicken broth, and a splash of almond milk.

- **Dinner:** Grilled shrimp skewers with cauliflower rice and steamed green beans.

- **Snack:** Sugar-free yogurt with mixed berries.

Day 6:

- **Breakfast:** Vanilla protein smoothie made with 1 scoop of protein powder, 1/2 banana, and 1 cup of unsweetened almond milk.

- **Lunch:** Pureed broccoli and cheddar cheese soup made with cooked broccoli, low-fat cheddar cheese, and vegetable broth.

- **Dinner:** Roasted chicken thigh with mashed cauliflower and sautéed kale.

- **Snack:** Sugar-free pudding cup.

Day 7:

- **Breakfast:** Greek yogurt with sliced peaches and a sprinkle of chopped almonds.

- **Lunch:** Creamy tomato and basil soup made with pureed tomatoes, basil, low-sodium chicken broth, and a splash of almond milk.

- **Dinner:** Baked turkey breast with roasted carrots and brown rice.

- **Snack:** Hard-boiled egg with a sprinkle of salt and pepper.

Week 4

Day 1:

- **Breakfast:** Protein smoothie made with 1 scoop of protein powder, 1/2 cup of mixed berries, and 1/2 cup of unsweetened almond milk.

- **Lunch:** Turkey and vegetable puree made with cooked turkey breast, mixed vegetables, and low-sodium chicken broth.

- **Dinner:** Baked salmon fillet with roasted asparagus and quinoa.

Snack: Cottage cheese with sliced peaches.

Day 2:

- **Breakfast:** Greek yogurt parfait with 1/2 cup of Greek yogurt, 1/4 cup of granola, and a handful of sliced strawberries.

- **Lunch:** Creamy cauliflower and cheese soup made with pureed cauliflower, low-fat cheese, and vegetable broth.

- **Dinner:** Grilled chicken breast with mashed sweet potatoes and steamed broccoli.

- **Snack:** Sugar-free gelatin with whipped cream.

Day 3:

- **Breakfast:** Diced bell peppers and onions with scrambled eggs.

- **Lunch:** Lentil and vegetable stew made with cooked lentils, diced tomatoes, onions, and vegetable broth.

- **Dinner:** Zucchini noodles served with turkey meatballs and marinara sauce.

- **Snack:** Protein shake made with 1 scoop of protein powder and 1/2 cup of unsweetened almond milk.

Day 4:

- **Breakfast:** Protein pancakes topped with sliced bananas and a drizzle of sugar-free syrup.

- **Lunch:** Creamy mushroom and thyme soup made with pureed mushrooms, thyme, low-sodium chicken broth, and a splash of almond milk.

- **Dinner:** Baked cod fillet with roasted Brussels sprouts and quinoa.

- **Snack:** Celery sticks with almond butter.

Day 5:

- **Breakfast:** Spinach and feta cheese omelette made with 2 eggs and a handful of spinach.

- **Lunch:** Creamy tomato and basil soup made with pureed tomatoes, basil, low-sodium chicken broth, and a splash of almond milk.

- **Dinner:** Grilled shrimp skewers with cauliflower rice and sautéed green beans.

- **Snack:** Sugar-free yogurt with mixed berries.

Day 6:

- **Breakfast:** Vanilla protein smoothie made with 1 scoop of protein powder, 1/2 banana, and 1 cup of unsweetened almond milk.

- **Lunch:** Pureed butternut squash soup made with roasted butternut squash, vegetable broth, and a splash of coconut milk.

- **Dinner:** Roasted chicken thigh with mashed cauliflower and steamed broccoli.

- **Snack:** Sugar-free pudding cup.

Day 7:

- **Breakfast:** Greek yogurt with sliced peaches and a sprinkle of chopped almonds.

- **Lunch:** Creamy broccoli and cheddar cheese soup made with pureed broccoli, low-fat cheddar cheese, and vegetable broth.

- **Dinner:** Baked turkey breast with roasted carrots and brown rice.

- **Snack:** Hard-boiled egg with a sprinkle of salt and pepper.

Chapter Thirteen

Tips for dining out

Dining out after gastric sleeve surgery can present some challenges, but with careful planning and consideration, it's entirely manageable. Here are some tips to help you navigate dining out:

- **Choose the Right Restaurant:** Look for restaurants that offer a variety of options, including lean proteins, vegetables, and soups. Avoid fast food or buffets where healthy options may be limited.

- **Review the Menu Ahead of Time:** A lot of restaurants now offer their menus online. Take advantage of this and review the menu before you go, so you can plan what to order in advance.

- **Focus on Protein:** Protein is essential for your recovery and for maintaining muscle mass after surgery. Look for dishes that are rich in lean protein, such as grilled chicken, fish, or tofu.

- **Watch Portion Sizes:** Restaurant portions tend to be larger than what you may need after surgery. Consider sharing a meal with a friend or asking for a smaller portion if available.

- **Avoid Liquid Calories:** Be cautious of high-calorie beverages like sugary sodas, alcoholic drinks, or creamy milkshakes. Stick to water, herbal tea, or unsweetened beverages to avoid consuming extra calories.

- **Choose Whole Foods:** Opt for dishes that are based on whole foods, such as grilled or steamed vegetables, salads with lean protein, and broth-based soups. Avoid dishes that are fried, breaded, or heavily processed.

- **Ask for Modifications:** Never be afraid to ask your waitress to make changes to accommodate your dietary requirements. Request grilled instead of fried, sauce on the side, or substitutions for healthier options.

- **Be Mindful of Texture:** In the early stages of recovery, you may still be adjusting to different textures of food. Choose softer options or meals that can be easily modified to a pureed or soft consistency if needed.

- **Listen to Your Body:** Pay attention to your body's hunger and fullness cues. Stop eating when you feel satisfied, even if there's food left on your plate.

- **Enjoy the Experience:** Dining out should be an enjoyable experience, so don't stress too much about making the perfect choice. Focus on spending time with friends or family and savoring the flavors of your meal.

By following these tips, you can make dining out after gastric sleeve surgery a positive and enjoyable experience while still prioritizing your health and nutritional needs.

Celebrating Your Gastric Sleeve Journey

Celebrating your gastric sleeve journey is an important part of your overall success and progress. Here are some ways you can celebrate your achievements:

- **Set Milestone Goals:** Celebrate reaching milestones along your journey, such as losing a certain amount of weight, fitting into a smaller clothing size, or achieving a health-related goal. Treat yourself to something special when you reach these milestones, whether it's a spa day, new workout gear, or a fun outing with friends.

- **Document Your Progress:** Take photos or keep a journal to document your progress throughout your gastric sleeve journey. Reflecting on how far you've come can be incredibly motivating and rewarding.

- **Share Your Success:** Share your success with friends, family, and your support network. Celebrate your achievements with loved ones who have been there for you throughout your journey.

- **Reward Yourself with Non-Food Treats:** Instead of celebrating with food, treat yourself to non-food rewards such as a new book, a movie night, a massage, or a new hobby or activity you've been wanting to try.

- **Celebrate NSVs (Non-Scale Victories):** Recognize and celebrate the non-scale victories that come with your gastric sleeve journey, such as improved energy levels, better sleep, increased mobility, and enhanced confidence.

- **Plan Special Activities:** Plan special activities or outings to celebrate your progress, such as a hike in nature, a day at the beach, or a weekend getaway to relax and recharge.

- **Join a Support Group:** Joining a support group of fellow gastric sleeve patients can provide a sense of community and camaraderie. Celebrate each other's successes and share tips and advice for navigating the journey together.

- **Practice Self-Care:** Take time to practice self-care and prioritize your physical and emotional well-being. Treat yourself to activities that promote relaxation and stress relief, such as meditation, yoga, or a bubble bath.

- **Reflect on Your Achievements:** Take time to reflect on how far you've come since undergoing gastric sleeve surgery. Celebrate your resilience, determination, and commitment to your health and well-being.

- **Celebrate Your New Lifestyle:** Embrace your new lifestyle and all the positive changes that come with it. Celebrate the healthier habits you've adopted and the positive impact they've had on your life.

Remember that celebrating your gastric sleeve journey is about acknowledging your hard work, perseverance, and dedication to improving your health and well-being. Celebrate both the big milestones and the small victories along the way, and continue to celebrate your progress as you journey towards a healthier and happier life.

Chapter Fourteen

Essential kitchen tools following gastric sleeve surgery

Having the right kitchen equipment is crucial for keeping a healthy lifestyle and accomplishing long-term weight loss objectives following bariatric surgery. The right kitchen equipment can ease the process of preparing meals, lessen stress when preparing, and offer convenience when attempting to maintain a balanced diet. Having the right tools in your kitchen can have a huge impact on how well you recover from surgery, from specialty cookware to appliances that make food preparation easier. The necessary essentials that any kitchen after bariatric surgery should have are listed below.

- **Blender:** A high-quality blender is crucial for preparing pureed foods, smoothies, and protein shakes during the early stages post-surgery.

- **Food Processor:** Useful for pureeing larger batches of food, chopping vegetables, and creating smooth textures for soups and sauces.

- **Immersion Blender:** Great for quickly blending soups directly in the pot, making it easier to achieve smooth, consistent textures.

- **Measuring Cups and Spoons:** Precise measurement of food portions is essential for maintaining portion control and tracking nutrient intake.

- **Kitchen Scale:** A digital kitchen scale helps you accurately measure food portions, which is important for monitoring intake and ensuring you stay within dietary guidelines.

- **Small Plates and Bowls:** Smaller dishware helps with portion control and makes it easier to manage smaller meals visually.

- **Slow Cooker or Instant Pot:** Ideal for preparing healthy, nutrient-dense meals with minimal effort. They're perfect for cooking lean meats and vegetables to tender perfection.

- **Steamer Basket:** Steaming is a healthy way to cook vegetables, fish, and other lean proteins while retaining their nutrients.

- **Non-Stick Cookware:** Non-stick pans and pots reduce the need for added fats like oil or butter when cooking, helping to keep meals lower in calories.

- **Protein Shaker Bottle:** Convenient for mixing protein shakes on-the-go, ensuring you can easily meet your protein requirements.

- **Portion Control Containers:** These help pre-measure meals and snacks, making it easier to stick to your dietary plan and avoid overeating.

- **Strainer/Sieve:** Useful for straining soups, sauces, and purees to achieve a smooth consistency, especially during the pureed and soft food stages.

- **Sharp Knives:** A good set of sharp knives makes food preparation quicker and safer, especially when cutting lean meats and fresh produce.

- **Storage Containers:** Having a variety of storage containers is essential for meal prepping and storing leftovers. Go for clear containers to easily identify contents.

- **Spice Grinder or Mortar and Pestle:** Enhancing the flavor of your meals without adding extra calories is key, and fresh spices can make a big difference.

Having these kitchen essentials will not only streamline meal preparation but also support your nutritional goals and overall success after gastric sleeve surgery.

Conclusion

The "Gastric Sleeve Bariatric Cookbook for Beginners" is a comprehensive cookbook created to assist you on your post-gastric sleeve journey. This cookbook provides a selection of recipes that have been specially created to accommodate the dietary restrictions and nutritional requirements of bariatric patients. Every dish has an emphasis on using foods that are high in protein, low in sugar, and high in nutrients to make sure that every meal promotes the best possible recovery and long-term health.

Beyond only offering recipes, the book also educates you on the value of mindful eating, portion control, and the progressive reintroduction of various food textures. With sections devoted to each phase of the diet progression following surgery—from clear liquids to solid foods—this cookbook is an invaluable and encouraging tool for managing the dietary challenges associated with gastric sleeve surgery.

Apart from providing useful advice, the "Gastric Sleeve Bariatric Cookbook for Beginners" encourages you to have a positive connection with food and enjoy your meals while making healthy choices. Because there is a recipe for every taste thanks to the variety, adopting a healthier lifestyle may be both fun and long-lasting. In the end, anyone looking to maintain their health and reach their weight loss objectives following bariatric surgery will find this cookbook to be an indispensable resource.

Measurement conversion

Dry Ingredient Conversions

3 teaspoons=1 tablespoon=1/2 ounce=14.3 grams
2 tablespoons=1/8 cup=1 fluid ounce=28.3 grams
4 tablespoons=1/4 cup=2 fluid ounces=56.7 grams
5 1/3 tablespoons=1/3 cup=2.6 fluid ounces=75.6 grams
8 tablespoons=1/2 cup=4 ounces=113.4 grams=1 stick butter
12 tablespoons=3/4 cup=6 ounces=.375 pound=170 grams
32 tablespoons=2 cups=16 ounces=1 pound=453.6 grams
64 tablespoons=4 cups=32 ounces=2 pounds=907 grams

Liquid Ingredient Conversions

1 cup=8 fluid ounces=1/2 pint=237 ml
2 cups=16 fluid ounces=1 pint=474 ml
4 cups=32 fluid ounces=1 quart=946 ml
2 pints=32 fluid ounces=1 quart=946 ml
4 quarts=128 fluid ounces=1 gallon=3.784 liters
8 quarts=one peck
4 pecks=one bushel
Dash=less than 1/4 teaspoon

Weight Ingredient conversions

1 ounce = 28 grams
1 pound = 16 ounces
1 pound = approximately 1/2 kilogram
1 kilogram = 1,000 grams
1 kilogram = 2.2 pounds

The dirty dozen and the clean fifteen

The Dirty Dozen

These are the twelve fruits and vegetables with the highest levels of pesticide residue, according to EWG's analysis. It's recommended to buy these organic whenever possible to reduce exposure to potentially harmful chemicals. The Dirty Dozen includes:

1. Strawberries
2. Spinach
3. Kale, collard and mustard greens
4. Peaches
5. Pears
6. Nectarines
7. Apples
8. Grapes
9. Bell and hot peppers
10. Cherries
11. Blueberries
12. Green beans

The Clean 15

These are the fifteen fruits and vegetables with the lowest levels of pesticide residue, making them safer options to buy conventionally grown. While buying organic is always beneficial, these items are less likely to contain significant pesticide residues. The Clean Fifteen includes:

1. Avocados
2. Sweet corn
3. Pineapples
4. Onions
5. Papayas
6. Sweet peas
7. Asparagus
8. Honeydew melons
9. Kiwi
10. Cabbage
11. Mushrooms
12. Mangoes
13. Sweet potatoes
14. Watermelon
15. Carrots